HUG A TREE

Plant a garden, smell the roses, brew a cup of chamomile tea—the green world offers many life-enhancing antidotes to the stresses of our fast-paced technological world.

In these pages, one of the world's leading herbalists offers green remedies from teas and tinctures to baths and aromas to soothe and uplift both body and mind. The following topics are covered:

- Anxiety
- Depression
- Insomnia
- Indigestion
- Hypertension
- Premenstrual Syndrome
- Stress and Children

ABOUT THE AUTHOR

As a member of Britain's National Institute of Medical Herbalists, David Hoffmann has been a phytotherapist for almost 20 years. He is Assistant Professor of Integral Health Studies at the California Institute of Integral Studies, is a founding member and past president of the American Herbalist Guild and was director of the California School of Herbal Studies. The author of nine books on herbalism, his second book, *The New Holistic Herbal*, has become a standard text and has been translated into eight languages. Mr. Hoffmann teaches phytotherapy at schools throughout the English-speaking world.

A KEATS GOOD HERB GUIDE

MEDICINE
21 CENTURY

HERBS TO RELIEVE STRESS

*Herbal approaches to relaxation and
natural easing of depression and anxiety*

David Hoffmann

Keats Publishing, Inc. ☿ New Canaan, Connecticut

Herbs to Relieve Stress is not intended as medical advice. intent is solely informational and educational. Please consult health professional should the need for one be indicated.

HERBS TO RELIEVE STRESS

Library of Congress Cataloging-in-Publication Data

Hoffmann, David, 1951–
    Herbs to relieve stress / David Hoffmann.
        p.   cm.
    Includes bibliographical references and index.
    ISBN 0-87983-758-6
    1. Stress management. 2. Herbs—Therapeutic use.
                        Title.
  RA785.H64   1996
  616.89—dc20   96-242
                                                              CI

Printed in the United States of America

Good Herb Guides are published by
Keats Publishing, Inc.
27 Pine Street (Box 876)
New Canaan, Connecticut 06840-0876

98 97 96   6 5 4 3 2 1

CONTENTS

GREEN STRESS MANAGEMENT

A profoundly stressful transformation is affecting all aspects of our culture, often manifesting as trauma, chaos, pain, disruption—the whole panoply of crises we are all too familiar with.

How to cope with the ever-mounting pressures on our lives in these crazy times? Much has been written about how to manage stress, and much of it contains valuable insights. However, it can be said that at the core of our personal and planetary challenges is the human experience of alienation, a profound spiritual "homesickness." Is there a way in which stress management programs can help us experience the elusive but nurturing sense of belonging?

Herbalism is the medicine of belonging, the direct experience of the whole healing the part. Our world blesses us with herbs, with leaves of life. In the face of humanity's blind abuse and rape of nature, we discover remedies that can help us survive the impact of our mistakes.

Herbalism abounds with opportunities to experience the reality of the healing presence of nature, whether in treating disease or in hugging a tree. Approaching herbalism from its array of diverse and divergent components illuminates a field of human endeavor that is a wonderful weaving of the miraculous and the mundane. It is a therapy that encompasses stimulating laxatives such as senna, the spiritual ecstasy of the Amazonian shaman and the beauty of the flower. The limits to what might be called the path of the herbalist are only those imposed by parochial vision and constipated imagination!

Herbalism offers the unique possibility of being introduced to our medicine. A bridge can be built between person and herb, enpowering the individual to be present and responsible in the healing process. A person can be given a packet of herb seeds, encouraging a direct experience of the life of the plant. This experience of herbal vitality will be translated into a deeper rapport with the impersonal medicine ingested. The patient will not only get the medical benefit from the herb but also the enlivening experience of growing and preparing his or her own healing. If there is no garden, part of the treatment might involve a window box.

Healing with herbal medicines is a unique and wonderful cooperation between humanity and the plants. This experience of wholeness is spirit in action, creating an opportunity for change and transformation. The plant world provides us with herbs that transform and enlighten, and also with plants that heal and nurture nerve tissue itself.

Orthodox medicine tends to reduce psychological problems to a biochemical level and assumes that "appropriate" drugs will sort out or at least hide the problem sufficiently to allow "normal" life to continue. Interestingly enough, some techniques in the field of complementary medicine assume or imply the other extreme: namely, that psychological factors are the cause of all disease. Treatment of the psyche is, therefore, the only appropriate way of healing and will take care of any physical problem. By bringing these two reductionist views together, we come closer to a holistic approach.

A holistic approach to healing acknowledges the interconnectedness of physiological and psychological factors, and regards the nervous system and its functions as a vital element in the treatment of the whole being. To be truly healthy, we have to take care of our physical health through the right diet and lifestyle, but we are also responsible for taking care of our emotional, mental and spiritual life. We should endeavor to live in a fulfilling, nurturing environment that supports emotional stability. Our thoughts should be creative and life-enhancing, open to the free flow of intuition and imagination, rather than conceptually rigid. And we should stay open to the free flow of the higher energies of our souls, without which health is impossible.

The whole therapy of herbalism is uniquely suited to treating nervous system problems and stress. From one perspective herbs are embodiments of energy and spirit, while from another they are packets of biochemicals. In fact they can be viewed as a reflection of the human mind/ brain itself! If used with awareness it is possible to address the needs of the human energy body as well the tissue involved. In fact, the complexities of the mind/body actually can help the herbalist select the correct remedy. Herbal medicine can be an ecologically and spiritually integrative tool—an ideal counterpart on the physical level for therapeutic techniques on the psychological level.

WHAT IS STRESS?

Stress is best described as a group of body-wide, non-specific responses induced by any number of situations or events. Just staying alive creates demands on the body for life-maintaining energy; even while we are asleep, our bodies continue to function. So by this definition, stress is a fundamental part of being alive and should not be avoided. The trick is to ensure that the degree of stress we experience is such that life is a joy, not a drag.

From this perspective, energy usage is one characteristic of stress. Another characteristic is lack of specificity. Any demands made upon us in daily life bring about certain reactions in the body. These same reactions occur under a whole range of different conditions, both physical and emotional—from hot and cold to joy and sorrow. As aware, feeling people, we probably make a big distinction between the pain caused by the loss of a loved one and the pain caused by the temperature dropping too fast; but the nature of the demand is unimportant at the biological level. To the body, it's all the same because the stress response is always the same. Nerve signals are sent from the brain to several glands, and these react by secreting hormones to cope with the task ahead. So stress is not just worry and strain. It is a keynote of life, with all its ups and downs. A new and exciting love can cause us as much stress as a cranky boss.

The wide array of triggers that elicit the stress response

are known as stressors. There are many potential stressors, such as: changes (vacation, marriage, divorce, a new job and so on); any intense emotion, such as fear or anger; fatigue, physical injury, surgery, temperature extremes, noise, crowding, illness.

Change is one of the most powerful stressors. Any kind of change in our lives, even one perceived as positive, requires an adaptation to a new set of circumstances. Getting married, getting divorced, entering college and graduating from college all require adaptation and thus are all stressors. The effects of stressors are cumulative. The more stressors in one's life at any given time, the higher the stress levels will be.

No two people are exactly alike as to which aspects of daily life will increase their stress levels. The identical life situation might be quite pleasant to one person while extremely stressful to another. In a general sense, a situation will be a stressor if it is perceived as threatening to well-being or requiring adjustment in any way. It is the perception of each situation that makes it either stressful or not, so almost any event or situation can be a stressor.

How Stress Contributes to Illness

There is a definite relationship between stress and illness. Although the exact nature of that relationship is not yet understood, a number of ideas have been suggested. Early theories tried to connect different illnesses with specific types of emotional conflict or personality and body types.

Hans Selye maintains that the biological reactions accompanying adaptation to stress result in both short- and long-term adverse physical changes. He calls these changes diseases of adaptation, since they are the outcome of a system of defenses against threatening stimuli. The disease process is thought to arise as a result of factors such as the physiological effect of certain hormones from the adrenal and pituitary glands, the impact of the inflammation process and a general state of lowered resistance. The actual disease that manifests itself depends on a range of factors, including genetics, physical weakness and even specifically learned bodily responses.

This helps explain the effects of life changes or events on health. Life changes require adjustments that might produce physiological reactions. Moreover, sustained and unsuccessful attempts at coping with change can eventually lower bodily resistance, thus enhancing the probability of illness. The more frequent and severe the life changes we experience, the more likely we are to become ill. As examples consider the following:

Heart disease. Stress contributes to heart disease in many ways. During periods of stress, the blood pressure rises and the pulse increases, placing an increased burden on the heart. Stress includes changes in blood chemistry, such as elevated cholesterol levels, that promote atherosclerosis. Finally, the coronary arteries that supply blood to the heart muscle itself narrow, reducing the amount of oxygen available to the heart muscle.

Infectious diseases. Excessive stress reduces the effectiveness of the immune response and thus increases the risk of infection. Many people find that they experience colds mostly during stressful periods. Similarly, both oral and genital herpes attacks tend to develop during periods of high stress.

Cancer. As with infectious diseases, excessive stress increases the risk of cancer by reducing the efficiency of the immune system. In every person, cells become cancerous from time to time. If the immune system is working properly, these cancerous cells are usually destroyed quickly.

Digestive disorders. The sympathetic nervous system, which is activated during periods of stress, reduces production of most digestive juices, except for stomach acid. Food lies in the stomach, the acid builds up in response to the presence of the food, causing indigestion. In time, this acid can erode the wall of the stomach or intestine, causing an ulcer. Indigestion is a very common sign of excessive stress. Further, many people overeat or undereat during stressful periods, contributing to weight-management problems.

Skin disorders. The impact of excessive stress on skin has long been recognized. Two very obvious effects are the appearance of rashes and premature aging. Stress produces rashes by modifying the activity of the immune mechanism. Premature aging of the skin results from stress-induced narrowing of the small blood vessels supplying food and oxygen to the skin cells.

STRESS AND HERBAL REMEDIES

Herbs can help the body and mind cope with the stress response in a number of ways, in addition to the rather simplistic ones of stimulation and relaxation. In Western herbalism today, it is common to differentiate between groups of herbs that have similar physiological effects on people. Herbs that act on the nervous system are collectively called *nervines,* and are grouped into nervine tonics, nervine relaxants and nervine stimulants. There are also muscle-relaxing antispasmodics and sleep-inducers known as *hypnotics.* Of most direct relevance for stress management are the *adaptogenic* herbs.

Adaptogens

As we approach the 21st century, we live in a world of stress, pollution, lack of meaning and lack of purpose. In the face of such a cultural alienation from nature, the plethora of diseases assailing the "civilized" world should come as no surprise. To heal these ills, the underlying causes must first be addressed and these causes are not only within the individual but within our culture as a whole. When a health problem is related to lowered resistance due to the impact of a hostile environment, we must first heal the hostile environment. In other words, even if there were a remedy that offered individuals protection against toxic chemicals, it would be preferable to remove the toxic chemical from the environment. This makes economic sense, is the right stance in Hippocratic terms and it is right action in spiritual terms.

When attention is given to appropriate support for the body under stressful conditions, nature comes to our rescue. Technically what is needed is an increase in nonspecific resistance to damaging man-made factors and illnesses. A range of herbal remedies are coming to light that do this. Soviet scientists coined the term 'adaptogens' to describe herbs that produce this wonderful increase in resistance and vitality, defining them like this:

- An adaptogen must show a non-specific activity, i.e., increase in power of resistance against physical, chemical or biological noxious agents.
- An adaptogen must have a normalizing influence independent of the nature of the pathological state.
- An adaptogen must be innocuous and must not influence normal body functions more than required.

In this sense adaptogens reinforce the nonspecific power of resistance against stressors, increase general capacities to withstand situations of stress, and hence guard against disease caused by overstress of the organism. The general aims of adaptogen treatment are a reduction of stress reactions during the alarm phase of the stress response, prevention or at least delaying of the state of exhaustion and hence a certain level of protection against long-term stress.

A number of herbs that can be described as adaptogens include **Ginseng, Siberian Ginseng, Ashwaganda, Shiitake** and **Schizandra**. It is worth looking at the evidence for adaptogenicity in a little depth. Rather than exploring the background for all these adaptogenic herbs we will focus on Siberian ginseng.

Siberian Ginseng (*Eleutherococcus senticosus*). Siberi
ginseng, one of the most remarkable of adaptogenic plan
has a wide range of uses and very low toxicity. There h
been a great deal of excellent clinical and laboratory r
search conducted in the Soviet Union, where Profess
Brehkman and his team have been studying the herb f
over 30 years. Largescale clinical trials have been unde
taken on both healthy and sick people with more th
1,000 published research papers devoted to its applicatic
the mechanism of action and investigation of its acti
principles.

Pharmacological research suggests that the active princ
ple of the adaptogenic plants—the *eleutherosides* from S
berian ginseng and the *panaxosides* from ginseng—a
saponin glycosides which increase the general nonspeci
resistance of the body to a whole range of diverse chem
cal, physical, psychological and biological factors.
safety and ability to increase the resistance of the norm
human body to extreme conditions make Siberian ginse
a remedy of great importance.

Studies on Siberian ginseng provide some of the b
clinical trials done on herbal medicines so far. Large nu
bers of people including control groups were involved
these studies. Between 1973 and 1975, 1,200 drivers fro
the Volga automobile plant were given 8 to 12 mg
Siberian ginseng extract daily with tea for two mont
each year in the spring and autumn. By the end of t
experiment illness among the drivers had *decreased* by
to 30 percent, while the total disease incidence amo
other workers at the plant *increased* by 20 percent. Bas
on these results, the authorities at the factory undertoo
mass program of preventive medicine with the herb in
winter of 1975. It was included in the diet as Siberi
ginseng sugar at a per day dose of 2 ml. Altogether, 13,0
persons were engaged in the experiment. The overall d
ease incidence dropped by 30 to 35 percent as compar
to a control group that did not use the remedy.

In another clinical trial a group of 54 miners received the extract before the beginning of their shift daily in June and July of 1976. The number of people reporting sick dropped by 33.3 percent and the number of days lost through illness by 45.6 percent. Reduction of the incidence of influenza and acute respiratory diseases was particularly impressive. In a strict medical sense, Siberian ginseng is an adrenal stimulant and not an antiviral remedy. However, the Russians have accumulated much data on the anti-influenzal effect of the herb as well. Such findings imply that either it possesses an invigorating and tonic action on natural immunity or it has direct antivirus activity.

Conditions shown to improve with Siberian ginseng. There is an ever-lengthening list of pathologies that have been demonstrated to improve with the use of this adaptogen. Here is a short list based on published results:

- Neurasthenia
- Hypertension
- Chronic gastritis
- Diabetes
- Atherosclerosis
- Tuberculosis
- Brain injuries
- Infectious disease

Cancer. Siberian ginseng is also being used in Russia for the post-operative treatment of cancer patients. Not only does it speed post-operative recovery, but it ameliorates the stress response that can aggravate metastasis, the spreading of cancer cells around the body. The ability of Siberian ginseng to potentiate antitumor immunity has also been discovered recently. It increases antineoplastic white blood cells (natural "killer cells") and induces the synthesis of γ-interferon by leukocytes. It is well known that stress decreases the activity of the immune system and

particularly that of the natural killer cells. An obviou
association exists here on a biochemical level betwee
stress, immune function and the herb Siberian ginseng.

In these times of pollution and exposure to strange an
dangerous chemicals, this fascinating plant may prove c
vital help as it also reduces the toxic impact of a numbe
of chemical compounds. In laboratory tests Siberian gir
seng was shown to decrease the sensitivity of mice an
rats to the toxicity of a range of chemicals. When th
animals were treated with cytotoxic drugs combined wit
Siberian ginseng, they lost less weight and their whit
blood count was higher than in the animals treated wit
the drugs alone. The implications for using this herb a
support in anticancer chemotherapy are clear and excitin

A fundamental problem with the use of cytotoxic drug
in cancer therapy is that not only do they destroy cance
cells, but healthy ones as well. In the test, lethal doses c
the drugs resulted in the animals' death, but when Siberia
ginseng, and drugs were used in combination, the deat
rate dropped. In a group of mice given thiophosphamid
in a dose of 16 mg/kg. 53 percent of the animals diec
After administering combined Siberian ginseng and thic
phosphamide only 15 percent of the animals died. Simila
results were obtained in a group of animals given ethym
din in a dose of 1.5 mg/kg. Thirty percent so treated diec
while all those receiving both herb and drug remaine
alive.

Siberian ginseng also appears able to reduce the narcoti
effects of a number of drugs. For example it shortens th
duration of sleep induced by sedatives. It may also prov
useful for prophylactic and therapeutic applications i
acute and chronic poisoning with some insecticides an
industrial poisons. This ability of Siberian ginseng
linked with its ability to activate the body's own metaboli
system for inactivating toxins. Therefore, Russian pharma
cologists advise the use of the extract in different dru
formulae to reduce their inherent toxicity.

* * *

It is clear that Siberian ginseng is a very special remedy indeed. It can increase individual resistance to the whole spectrum of factors that contribute to stress reactions and exhaustion. Apparently the herb will help whether the stress is from extremes of weather or from psychological exhaustion. Its universal properties make this herb one of the most efficacious and promising medicines for increasing hardiness against the many stresses of contemporary life.

Nervines

A nervine is a plant that has an effect upon the nervous system in some way: there are nervine tonics, nervine relaxants and nervine stimulants. Remember that any successful treatment of nervous system problems with herbs must involve treating the whole body, heart and mind, not simply the signs of agitation and worry. Of course, the agitation can be reduced greatly by the appropriate herbs, but the whole system must be strengthened in the face of the storm as well.

Nervine tonics. Perhaps the most helpful contribution herbal medicine can make is to strengthen and "feed" the nervous system. In cases of shock, stress or nervous debility, the nervine tonics strengthen and restore the tissues directly. On the other hand they can contribute to the healing of damaged nervous tissue, whether this is due to a pathological process or physical trauma. This invaluable group of remedies is best exemplified by **oats**. **Ginkgo** is an important tonic for the nervous system, but appears to work via its vasodilating action on the blood vessels of the brain, thereby increasing oxygen availability to brain cells. Other nervine tonics can have, in addition, a relaxing effect. **Skullcap** is often the most effective, particularly for problems related to stress.

Mild relaxing nervines		
Balm	Chamomile	Lavender
Black cohosh	Hyssop	Red clover
Medium relaxing nervines		
Damiana	Motherwort	Skullcap
Linden	Mugwort	St. John's Wort
Lobelia	Pulsatilla	Vervain
Strong relaxing nervines		
California poppy	Passionflower	Wild lettuce
Hops	Valerian	

Nervine relaxants. This group of nervines are extremely useful in our times of stress and confusion, alleviating many of the accompanying symptoms. They should always be used in a broad holistic way, not simply to tranquilize. Too much tranquilizing, even that achieved through herbal medication, can in time deplete and weigh heavily on the whole nervous system.

Many of the nervine relaxants also have other properties and can be selected to aid in related problems. This is one of the great benefits of using herbal remedies to help in stress and anxiety problems. The physical symptoms that often accompany anxiety may be treated with herbs that work on the anxiety itself. They can also be grouped in terms of their relative strength, bearing in mind that not all people respond to herbs in the same way.

Since each system of the body has plants that are particularly suited to it, relaxing nervines can be selected based on their affinity for the various systems.

• *Circulatory system:* **Balm**, **linden** and **motherwort** are generally helpful to the cardiovascular system. However, most remedies that reduce overactivity in the nervous system will aid the heart and ameliorate problems such as high blood pressure.

- *Respiratory system:* Most sedatives will help in asthma, but **black cohosh, lobelia, motherwort** and **wild lettuce** are especially helpful.
- *Digestive system:* All the relaxing and antispasmodic remedies may be of value here to ease colic, but sedatives that actively aid digestion include **balm, chamomile** and **lavender.**
- *Reproductive system:* **Black cohosh, blue cohosh, crampbark, motherwort** and **wild lettuce** all have an affinity for this system.
- *Muscles and skeleton:* All sedative remedies will ease muscular tension and thus pain in this complex system. **Black cohosh** is especially helpful.
- *Nervous system:* All the remedies mentioned above relate here.
- *Skin:* All these nervines may help the skin in an indirect way, but the following herbs are especially beneficial for the skin: **red clover, St. John's wort, pulsatilla** and **black cohosh.**

While any of the above nervines will be generally relaxing, another way to select the herb (or herbs) that will prove most appropriate is to take into account their other properties. The range of options and the various subtleties can be daunting and complex, but as examples consider the list below. It combines the need for relaxation with other common symptoms as an indication for relevant herbs.

- *Delayed menstruation:* **black cohosh, motherwort,** mugwort.
- *Diarrhea:* **black haw, crampbark, hops, linden.**
- *Muscle tightness:* **black cohosh, black haw, crampbark, hops, lavender, lobelia, valerian.**
- *Colic:* **balm, black haw, chamomile, hops, hyssop, lavender, linden, mugwort, valerian.**
- *Sinus congestion:* **chamomile, hyssop, linden.**
- *Heartburn:* **balm, chamomile, linden.**
- *Arthritis:* **black cohosh, Jamaican dogwood.**
- *Skin problems:* **red clover.**

- *Flatulence:* **balm, chamomile, hops, hyssop, lavender, motherwort, mugwort, valerian.**
- *Hypertension:* **linden, motherwort, passionflower, scullcap, valerian.**
- *Asthma:* **lobelia, motherwort, wild cherry bark, wild lettuce.**
- *Menstrual cramps:* **black cohosh, blue cohosh, crampbark, motherwort, skullcap, valerian, wild lettuce.**

Nervine stimulants. Direct stimulation of the nervous tissue is not often needed in our times of hyperactivity. It is usually more appropriate to stimulate the body's innate vitality with the help of nervine or bitter tonics, which work by augmenting bodily harmony and thus have a much deeper and longer-lasting effect than nervine stimulants. In the last century much more emphasis was placed by herbalists upon stimulant herbs. It is, perhaps, a sign of the times that our world is supplying us with more than enough stimulus.

When direct nervine stimulation is indicated, an herb to use is **kola nut**, although **guarana, coffee, maté,** and **tea** should also be remembered. A problem with these commonly used stimulants is that they have a number of side effects and can themselves be involved in aggravating psychological problems such as anxiety and tension.

Some of the herbs rich in volatile oils are also valuable stimulants; among them the commonest and best are **rosemary** and **peppermint.**

Antispasmodics

In addition to the herbs that work directly on the nervous system, the antispasmodic herbs—which affect the peripheral nerves and the muscle tissue—can have an indirect relaxing effect on the body. When the physical body is at ease, a relaxed psyche follows. Many of the nervine relaxants have

Antispasmodics			
Balm	Californian poppy	Crampbark	Hyssop
Black cohosh	Catmint	Damiana	Jamaican dogwood
Black haw	Celery seed	Ginger	Lavender
Bugleweed	Chamomile	Hops	Linden
Licorice	Pasque flower	Skullcap	Vervain
Lobelia	Passionflower	Skunk cabbage	Wild cherry
Motherwort	Peppermint	St. John's wort	Wild lettuce
Mugwort	Red clover	Sundew	Wild yam
Mullein	Roman chamomile	Thyme	
Parsley	Rosemary	Valerian	

this antispasmodic action. The antispasmodics relax the autonomic nervous system and not necessarily the central nervous system. This allows a physical relaxation of muscles without a sedative effect upon consciousness.

Listed below are some common conditions and the appropriate antispasmodic herbs for relieving them:

- *Delayed menstruation:* **black cohosh, caraway, motherwort, mugwort, pennyroyal.**
- *Diarrhea:* **black haw, bugleweed, crampbark, ground ivy, hops, linden, red sage, rosemary, St. John's wort, wild cherry.**
- *Muscle tightness:* **black cohosh, black haw, crampbark, hops, lavender, lobelia, valerian.**
- *Colic:* **angelica, aniseed, balm, caraway, cardamom, catnip, chamomile, dill, fennel, fenugreek, ginger, hops, hyssop, lavender, motherwort, mug-**

wort, parsley, pennyroyal, peppermint, red sage, Roman chamomile, rosemary, thyme, valerian, vervain, wild carrot.

- *Sinus congestion:* betony, catmint, chamomile, coltsfoot, elder, fenugreek, ginger, hyssop, lavender, linden, mullein, peppermint, red sage, thyme
- *Heartburn:* coltsfoot, fenugreek, licorice, mullein.
- *Arthritis:* angelica, black cohosh, celery seed, elder, lavender, linden, licorice, wild yam.
- *Skin problems:* black cohosh, red clover.
- *Flatulence:* balm, chamomile, hops, hyssop, lavender, motherwort, mugwort, valerian.
- *Hypertension:* linden, motherwort, passionflower, scullcap, valerian.
- *Asthma:* lobelia, motherwort, wild cherry bark, wild lettuce.
- *Menstrual cramps:* black cohosh, black haw, crampbark, motherwort, skullcap, valerian, wild lettuce.

Hypnotics

Hypnotics are herbal remedies that will help to induce a deep and healing state of sleep. They have nothing at all to do with hypnotic trances. Herbs that promote sleep have modes of action that vary from mild, muscle-relaxing properties through volatile oils that ease psychological tensions to remedies that contain strong alkaloids that work directly on the central nervous system and put you to sleep. Some of the most effective plant hypnotics are illegal for the very reason of their effectiveness. This includes the whole range of opium poppy derivatives. The remedies mentioned here are entirely safe and have no addictive properties. When treating sleep problems, hypnotic herbs should always be used in conjunction with attention to relaxation diet and lifestyle.

Each system of the body has plants that are particularly suited to it, some of which are hypnotics of varying

Mild hypnotics
Mugwort   Chamomile   Linden

Medium hypnotics
California   Motherwort   Pulsatilla   Skullcap
  poppy

Strong hypnotics
Hops   Passionflower Wild lettuce
Jamaican   Valerian
  dogwood

strength. It is safe to say, however, that all the hypnotic remedies can help the whole body in that sleep is such a vital health process.

- *Circulatory system:* **Motherwort, linden, balm.** Notice that they are all in the milder group.
- *Respiratory system:* All of the hypnotics can help as antispasmodics in conditions such as asthma, if used at the right dose. **Wild lettuce** eases irritable coughs.
- *Digestive system:* The relaxing nervines and carminatives are important, especially **chamomile, balm, hops** and **valerian.** The antispasmodic herbs will help with intestinal colic, for example, **hops, Jamaican dogwood, passionflower** and **valerian.**
- *Muscles and skeleton:* All hypnotics will aid in reducing muscle tension and even the pain associated with problems in this system. They may be used internally or as lotions. Especially important are **Jamaican dogwood** and **valerian.**
- *Skin:* **Chamomile** and **cowslip** are healing, but otherwise the value of hypnotics here is to ensure that the body has a good recuperative rest each night.

Bach Flower Remedies

This unique healing system consists of essences made from 38 different flowers, each having a specific action upon a certain mental attitude. Just as the body has its own self-healing properties regarding diseases and wounds, the mind and spirit have their own self-healing capacities, which the Bach Flower Remedies stimulate. The remedies used are all prepared from the flowers of wild plants, bushes and trees, and none of them is harmful or habit-forming.

They are used for worry, apprehension, hopelessness, irritability and so on, because these states of mind or moods hinder recovery of health, retard convalescence and often are the underlying causes of sickness and disease. A long-continued worry or fear depletes one's vitality.

It is important to identify the nature of the individual's unique "patterns" before selecting the appropriate remedy. Consider the person's attitudes, feelings, worries, indecision, timidity, vexations, resentment, possessiveness, hopelessness, lethargy, hatred, overpowering or demanding nature, intolerance, tenseness, etc. and, most importantly, the reason behind the apprehension, worry and fear. Only then can the correct remedy or remedies be determined.

- AGRIMONY. Those who suffer inner torture which they try to hide behind a facade of cheerfulness. Often used as a remedy for alcoholism.
- ASPEN. Apprehension, the feeling that something dreadful is going to happen without knowing why. Anxiety for no known reason.
- BEECH. Critical and intolerant of others. Arrogant.
- CENTAURY. Weakness of will; those who let themselves be exploited or imposed upon; they have difficulty in saying "no." A human doormat.
- CERATO. Those who doubt their own judgment and intuition, always seeking the advice of others. Often influenced and misguided.

- CHERRY PLUM. Uncontrolled, irrational thoughts. Fear of losing control and doing something terrible, fear of "going crazy." Uncontrolled bursts of temper. Impulsively suicidal.
- CHESTNUT BUD. Refusal to learn by experience; continually repeating the same mistakes.
- CHICORY. Overly possessive, demands respect or attention, likes others to conform to their standards. Makes martyr of oneself. Interferes and manipulates.
- CLEMATIS. Indifferent, inattentive, daydreaming, absent-minded. Mental escapist from reality.
- CRAB APPLE. "The Cleanser Flower." Feels unclean or ashamed of ailments. Self disgust/hatred. House proud.
- ELM. Temporarily overcome by inadequacy or responsibility, though normally very capable.
- GENTIAN. Despondent. Easily discouraged and rejected. Skeptical, pessimistic. Depression when the cause is known.
- GORSE. Desperate, without hope: "Oh, what's the use?" Defeatism.
- HEATHER. People who are obsessed with their own troubles and experiences. Talkative bores, poor listeners.
- HOLLY. For those who are jealous, envious, revengeful and suspicious. Those who hate.
- HONEYSUCKLE. For those with nostalgia who constantly dwell in the past. Homesickness.
- HORNBEAM. "Monday morning" feeling but once started, task is usually fulfilled. Mentally tired. Procrastination.
- IMPATIENS. Impatience, irritability. Reacts in an exaggerated manner.
- LARCH. Despondency due to lack of self-confidence; expectation of failure, so fails to make the attempt. Feels inferior, yet has the ability.
- MIMULUS. Fear of known things, fear of the world. Shyness, timidity, bashfulness.

- MUSTARD. Dark cloud of depression that descends for no known reason which can lift just as suddenly, making one downcast, saddened and low.
- OAK. Brave determined type. Struggles on in illness and against adversity despite setbacks. Plodders, never resting.
- OLIVE. Drained of energy, everything an effort. Physically fatigued.
- PINE. Feelings of guilt. Blames oneself for the mistakes of others. Feels unworthy.
- RED CHESTNUT. Excessive care of and concern for others, especially those held dear.
- ROCK ROSE. Alarmed, panicky, full of trepidation.
- ROCK WATER. For those who are hard on themselves and often overwork. Rigid, self-denying, ascetic.
- SCLERANTHUS. Uncertainty, indecision, vacillation. Fluctuating moods.
- STAR OF BETHLEHEM. For all the effects of upsetting news or fright following an accident. For release from trauma, no matter how old it is.
- SWEET CHESTNUT. Absolute dejection. Feels as if one has reached the limits of what one can stand.
- VERVAIN. Over-enthusiasm, over effort, straining. Fanatical and highly strung. Incensed and frustrated by injustices.
- VINE. Dominating/inflexible/ambitious/tyrannical/autocratic. Arrogant pride. Considered to be good leaders.
- WALNUT. Protection remedy against powerful influences; helps adjustment to any transition or change, e.g., puberty, menopause, divorce, new surroundings. Unlike Centaury the person knows what he wants, but is easily influenced by other people to do something else.
- WATER VIOLET. Proud, reserved, sedate types, sometimes feel "superior." Little emotional involvement, but reliable, dependable.

- WHITE CHESTNUT. Persistent unwanted thoughts. Preoccupation with some worry or episode. Mental arguments. Constant inner dialogue.
- WILD OAT. Helps determine one's intended path of life.
- WILD ROSE. Resignation, apathy. Drifters who accept their lot, making little or no effort for improvement; lacks ambition.
- WILLOW. Resentment and bitterness with "not fair" and "poor me" attitude.

* * *

- RESCUE REMEDY. Dr. Bach combined five specific Remedies (Cherry Plum, Clematis, Impatiens, Rock Rose, Star of Betlehem) to formulate an emergency composite that he called Rescue Remedy. Its purpose is to comfort, reassure and calm those who have received upsetting news or have experienced a trauma. Rescue Remedy is invaluable to keep at hand for immediate emergency use; however it does not take the place of medical attention. It is taken orally (4 drops in a glass of water), but can also be applied externally either in liquid or cream form.

The Bach Remedies are benign in their action without unpleasant side effects; thus, they can be taken by anyone. Stock concentrate remedies will keep indefinitely; a 10 ml concentrate bottle will make approximately 60 treatment bottles. More than one remedy can be taken at the same time. Place 2 drops of each chosen remedy in a glass of water and sip at intervals during the day or prepare a treatment bottle: fill a 1 fl. oz dropper bottle with spring water, add 2 drops of each chosen remedy and place 4 drops of this mixture directly on the tongue at least 4 times a day.

THE ROLE OF HERBS IN STRESS MANAGEMENT

A well-balanced stress management program must address all aspects of life, and while herbal remedies will only fulfill some aspects, they are vital. It can help to group the many factors to be considered into four categories.

1. **Physiological and metabolic factors.** This involves addressing factors affecting the inner workings of the body through nutrition, herbs and drugs, when necessary. Herbal medicines offer an effective but gentle way to address some of the physiological and biochemical issues involved in stress management ranging from direct support of the adrenal glands to easing the plethora of symptoms that can result from the stress response.

2. **Structural factors.** Here techniques are considered that address structural integration. This includes the manipulative therapies such as osteopathy, chiropractic and all varieties of massage. Personal lifestyle will contribute exercise, dance or any expression of bodily vitality. Relaxation techniques are invaluable.

3. **Emotional and mental factors.** Psychological techniques are important for identifying and treating emotional and mental factors in health and disease. All the branches of psychotherapy are involved here, but especially the more holistically oriented approaches of humanistic and transpersonal psychology. A conscious and free-flowing emotional life is fundamental to achieving any inner harmony. This does not mean that everyone must get involved in depth psychology, but that attention be given in the appropriate form for an individual's emotional needs.

4. **Spirituality.** Spiritual factors in human healing are becoming increasingly recognized by materialistic Western medicine. There are meditative and prayer-based techniques where the person aligns his or her being with a higher spirit, or those where a practitioner works with the energy body of a patient. Some openness to spirituality is vital and it might take the form of an uplifting sunset, being touched by poetry or art, belief in a religion or simply joy in being alive.

Gardening, Tree Hugging and Stress Management

If we get a bit creative it is easy to see how herbalism fits into a broad holistic context. The role of herbs need not be limited to their ingestion. This is a perfect excuse to get into the garden, walk in the woods and literally "smell the roses!"

As we shall see later in the book chamomile is a very useful relaxing herb, combining a pleasant flavor with a range of relevant properties. Before the Victorians developed the grass lawn (a major cause of stress for some people!) lawns were made up of varieties of herbs that could cope with being trampled upon, and chamomile was one of these. A chamomile lawn makes a wonderfully restful place where you can lie on the herbs, relaxing the body while the wonderful aroma wafts around you. If the lawn is one you grew yourself there are the added stress-reducers of exercise and a sense of fulfillment.

A specific variety of chamomile must be used: *Chamoemelum nobile*, "Treneague," is an apple-scented, non-flowering variety which works well, but the ordinary Roman chamomile saved from seed, which is less expensive, can also be used. Prepare the soil and then broadcast the seed. Cover with a thin layer of soil and keep moist but not wet. Once seedlings appear and have at least two sets of leaves, thin them out to about three inches apart. Don't walk on them until they are beginning to bind together. Remove most flower heads as they appear to ensure leaf vigor, but allow occasional flowers to remain as they form part of the lawn's charm. Avoid having a chamomile lawn bordering on a grass or wild garden area as creeping weeds will soon invade the lawn, and uprooting them will disturb the shallow-rooted chamomile plants. A surround of stone, brick or paving slabs is ideal.

If a very broad view is taken of herbalism, seeing it as an exploration of humanity's relationship with the plant world, some unusual healing possibilities present themselves. In recent years, researchers from several disciplines have begun investigating the benefits of contacts with plants, especially trees. In studies of the stress-reducing effects of nature, people recovered more quickly and completely from stress when exposed to plant-rich natural settings. This was indicated by lower blood pressure, heart rate, muscle tension, and skin conductance. Psychological recovery was also facilitated with measurable reductions of fear and anger and increases in positive feelings. Physiological findings indicated that the nature settings produced significant recovery from stress in only four to six minutes. This rapid recovery highlights the importance of plants for city dwellers who are often stressed out by commuting and work pressures.

In a comparison of the hospital records of gall bladder surgery patients who had window views of either a small stand of trees or a brick building wall, it was found that those with the view of trees had shorter postoperative hospital stays, required fewer potent drugs for pain and received fewer negative staff evaluations about their conditions than those with the wall view.

In a comparison of the free-fall behavior of ball bearings on the 40th-story window ledge of different heights...

HERBAL TREATMENTS FOR STRESS

Anxiety

When the level of stress goes beyond the point of being a healthy stimulant and starts to adversely affect our health, it often takes the form of anxiety. It might surface as fear, apprehension, or a wide range of bodily symptoms. These are most prominent in the early stages of the illness and represent a reasonable reaction to the onset of illness and the related uncertainties.

Generalized anxiety disorder (GAD) is much more than the normal anxiety people experience day to day. It is chronic and exaggerated worry and tension, even though nothing seems to provoke it. Having this disorder means always anticipating disaster, often worrying excessively about health, money, family or work. Sometimes, though, the source of the worry is hard to pinpoint. Simply the thought of getting through the day might provoke anxiety. People with GAD can't seem to shake their concerns, even though they usually realize that their anxiety is more intense than the situation warrants. They also seem unable to relax and have trouble falling or staying asleep. Their worries are accompanied by any of the physical symptoms listed on the following pages.

There may be no recognizable basis for the fear or feeling of threat, or the actual stimulus may be completely out of proportion to the emotion it provokes. Nevertheless, the symptoms it provokes are very real. For some people, anxiety takes the form of recurrent attacks that, though they occur unpredictably, may become associated with specific situations. They start with a sudden, intense apprehension, often combined with a feeling of impending doom and sometimes with feelings of unreality. Any of the symptoms described below may occur. An "anticipatory fear" or loss of control often develops, so that the person experiencing the attack becomes afraid of, for example, being left alone in a public place. The anticipatory fear may itself precipitate other symptoms that escalate the attack.

People with panic disorder have feelings of terror that strike suddenly and repeatedly with no warning. They can't predict when an attack will occur, and many develop intense anxiety between episodes, worrying when and where the next one will strike. In between times there is a persistent, lingering worry that another attack could come any minute. While most attacks average a couple of minutes, occasionally they can go on for up to 10 minutes. In rare cases, they may last an hour or more.

SYMPTOMS OF ANXIETY. There are a whole range of reactions associated with anxiety.*

Anxious mood: Worrying, apprehension, anticipation of the worst, irritability.

The remedies: The herbal approaches described in the following section will be generally helpful, but the Bach Flower Remedies are especially relevant. For example

*Adapted from: Hamilton, M. "The Assessment of Anxiety States by Rating," British Journal of Medical Psychology, 32, 1959, pp 50-55.

aspen and **rock rose** are indicated in states of apprehension.

Fear: Of the dark, being left alone, traffic, strangers, large animals, crowds.

The remedies: Again it is the Bach Flower Remedies that shine here, especially **cherry plum** and **mimulus.**

Cognitive symptoms: Difficulty in concentration, poor memory.

The remedies: The specifics suggested for stress management given in the following pages are indicated with the possible addition of **ginkgo** and **rosemary** to help with difficulty in concentration and poor memory. **Basil** essential oil can be used to aid concentration as an inhalation. A 'brain tonic' tea can easily be made to increase memory and improve the ability to concentrate. Mix the following herbs and infuse 1-2 teaspoonfuls of the mixture in a cup of boiling water for 10-15 minutes. Drink 3 times a day:

- Rosemary, 1 part
- Ginkgo leaves, 4 parts
- Yerba maté, 1 part
- Gota kola, 2 parts

Depressed mood: Loss of interest, depression, diurnal mood swings. Lack of pleasure in hobbies, early waking.

The remedies. In addition to the herbal suggestions that follow, the Bach Flower Remedies can be especially relevant. Consider **gentian, gorse, mustard, olive, sweet chestnut** and **wild rose.**

General body sensations: Tinnitus, hot and cold flushes prickling sensations, blurred vision, feelings of weakness

The remedies. All of the relaxing nervines and relaxing exercises will ease this group of symptoms.

Respiratory symptoms: Pressure or constriction in chest tightness of breath, feelings of choking, sighing.

The remedies. All of the relaxing nervines and relaxing exercises will ease this group of symptoms.

Genitourinary symptoms: Frequency in urination, suppressed menstrual periods, frigidity, premature ejaculation, impotence, urgency of urination, excessive bleeding during period, loss of erection.

The remedies. These symptoms can be treated with herbal medicines that are not directly relevant to the topic of stress management. This highlights the need for competent diagnosis to ensure appropriate treatment. See *Herbs for Women's Health* by Mary Bove, N.D. and Linda Costarella, N.D. and *Herbs for Men's Health* by CJ Puotinen (Keats Publishing, Inc.).

Physiological symptoms. Tremor of hands, strained face, swallowing, sweating, furrowed brow, facial pallor, belching, eyelid twitching.

The remedies: All of the antispasmodics, relaxing nervines and relaxing exercises will ease this group of symptoms.

Tension. Feelings of tension, inability to relax, easily moved to tears, feelings of restlessness, fatigue, startled response, trembling.

The remedies. Again the relaxing nervines and relaxing exercises will help but in addition the essential oils of **lavender** and **rose geranium** are especially helpful. The Bach Flower Remedies **hornbeam, olive** and **rock rose** should also be considered.

Insomnia: Difficulty in falling asleep, unsatisfying sleep, fatigue on waking, night terrors, broken sleep, dreams, nightmares.

The remedies. Herbal approaches are discussed on page 37.

General somatic symptoms: Muscular aches and pains, muscular twitching, muscular stiffness, grinding teeth.

The remedies. Muscle relaxing antispasmodics such as **crampbark** and the stronger relaxing nervines such as **valerian** are effective here.

Cardiovascular symptoms: Tachycardia, chest pain, feelings of faintness, palpitations, throbbing of blood vessels, skipped heartbeats.

The remedies. Herbal medicine has much to offer for the gentle treatment of heart problems in this body system and are discussed in *Herbs for the Heart* by CJ Puotinen (Keats Publishing, Inc.).

Gastrointestinal symptoms: Difficulty in swallowing, indigestion, heartburn, looseness of bowels, constipation, gas, burps, bloating, weight loss.

The remedies. One of the strengths of herbal medicine is its efficacy in the treatment of digestive system problems, and especially those that are stress-related. This is discussed below and in much more depth in *Herbs to Improve Digestion* by CJ Puotinen (Keats Publishing, Inc.).

Autonomic nervous system symptoms: Dry mouth, pallor, giddiness, flushing, tendency to sweat.

The remedies. All of the relaxing nervines and relaxing exercises will ease this group of symptoms.

Managing Stress

If a period of stress is predictably about to occur, it can be prepared for ahead of time, as herbs, diet and any appropriate lifestyle changes will minimize the impact. Nervine relaxants can be used regularly as gentle soothing remedies. The following herbs can be taken as teas, cold drinks, infused in massage oil, used in relaxing foot baths or full baths.

- Balm
- Chamomile
- Lavender
- Linden
- Mugwort
- Oats
- Red Clover
- Skullcap
- St. John's Wort

A daily supplement of the B-complex vitamins and vitamin C is also suggested. By using herbs and improving the diet, you are responding to stress in a healthy way, and the impact of the various stressors can be ameliorated. Relaxation exercises and an honest reevaluation of both lifestyle and life-goals are invaluable. This is not always easy, but remember that people can change, change their lives and reevaluate their choices.

The line between chronic stress and the daily levels we all seem to put up with is fuzzy. A gentle soul with a delicate constitution will cross the line sooner than a stronger person who copes well. Neither of these extremes is better than the other; they merely reflect the fact that we live in a world of human diversity. That's sometimes a joy and sometimes an actual cause of stress! The advice given above holds for chronic stress, but in addition, adaptogens become pivotal in this situation. Important examples are **ginseng**, **Siberian ginseng** and **ashwaganda.**

Perhaps **Siberian ginseng** is the most highly recommended because it has no toxicity and lacks the stimulating effects some people experience with **Korean** or **American ginseng.** The usual dosage of the tincture is ½-¾ tsp. three times a day. Commercial products are increasingly made from a highly concentrated dry extract. First they are extracted using a liquid which is dried to a powder and then made into tablets. An equivalent dosage using a solid extract concentrated at a ratio of 20:1 would be 100-200 mg. The recommended regime is usually for a 6-week course followed by a 2-week break. This regime can be repeated for as long as is necessary.

In addition to adaptogens, every attention must be given

to general health as the body will often show its stress through some physical symptom. This may be a long-standing complaint that gets worse, an old problem that reappears or just a speeding of the aging process.

There are times in most people's lives when things get to be too much and the pain of existence builds to a crescendo. Immediate herbal relief may be needed in a whole range of traumatic situations—from being involved in a car accident to some personal emotional crisis. In all cases, herbs will take the edge off the trauma but will rarely remove it. At such times herbs can be only an aid, just one element of the approach taken to deal with the difficulties being faced. This approach may also include seeking help from a health professional, going on vacation or a retreat or even checking into a hospital.

The plants that are capable of easing intense stress are considered dangerous in our society and because they are restricted drugs, they will not be discussed here. However, in addition to the herbs previously mentioned, the following remedies might be considered: **passionflower, valerian, wild lettuce.**

Basic Stress Formula

> Skullcap 2 parts
> Valerian 2 parts
> Oats 1 part
> Take 1 tsp. tincture as needed.

Notice the dosage here (1 tsp. of tincture as needed). This is a recognition that the stress response has a cyclical nature and each person will find certain times of the day more challenging than others. As this is largely symptomatic medication, it may be increased until the desired relief is experienced. The dosage regime may be altered as necessary, varying time of day and quantity of dose to suit individual needs. For example, this may be a large dose first thing in the morning, or smaller amounts at frequent intervals throughout the day. The patient's experience is the guiding principle here. Always treat the human being and not the theory about the disease.

A possible prescription for acute stress associated with indigestion and palpitations:

Skullcap 2 parts
Valerian 2 parts
Motherwort 1 part
Chamomile 1 part
Mugwort 1 part
Take 1 tsp of tincture as needed.

The motherwort supports relaxation but also has a specific calming impact on palpitations.

Depression

Depression is a state of mind familiar to almost everyone, but this very familiarity becomes problematic when approaching clinical depressive states. In ordinary usage the word refers to a mood state that in medicine is called *dysthemia,* as contrasted with the normal state of *euthymia* and the opposite state of elation. In psychiatric usage, disorders of mood are called affective disorders; depression can be such a disease in itself or a symptom of another mental disorder. Normal human responses to some situations may also include transient depressions.

Major depression occurs in 10 percent to 20 percent of the world's population in the course of a lifetime. Women are more often affected than men, by a two-to-one ratio, and they seem to be at particular risk in the period prior to menstruation or following childbirth. Relatives of patients with major depression also seem to be at some higher risk of becoming depressed, and about 2 percent of the population may have a chronic disorder known as a depressive personality.

Depression is defined by a standard set of symptoms

described in the American Psychiatric Association's Diagnostic and Statistical Manual of Mental Disorders. They are:

- Poor appetite and significant weight loss, or increased appetite and significant weight gain.
- Insomnia or increased sleep.
- Agitation or retardation of movement and thought.
- Loss of interest or pleasure in usual activities or decrease in sexual drive.
- Fatigue and loss of energy.
- Feelings of worthlessness, self-reproach or excessive or inappropriate guilt.
- Diminished ability to think or concentrate; indecisiveness.
- Recurrent thoughts of death or suicide; or suicide attempts.

Not all of these characteristics occur in each individual who becomes depressed. For purposes of psychiatric treatment, a person is considered to have experienced a major depressive episode if he or she exhibits a loss of interest or pleasure in all or almost all usual activities and shows at least four of the above symptoms nearly every day for a period of at least two weeks. The term depression is often modified by words that imply either some specific factor or some chemical mechanism is the cause of the state.

- Depressions that are reactions to some loss of or separation from a valued person or object are called reactive (or exogenous) depressions.
- This contrasts with the usually more severe depressions without apparent cause, called endogenous depressions, or those accompanied by delusions.

Specific remedies for depression

St. John's wort (*hypericum*) has a long tradition of use in Europe, and while it sometimes gets remarkable results it is also sometimes ineffective. It takes time to work, so it must be taken for at least a month.

A double-blind, clinical trial was conducted in 1993 testing the antidepressant effects of St. John's wort extract. One hundred and five out-patients with depressions of short duration were treated in a double-blind study either with 300 mg of St. John's wort extract 3 times a day or with a placebo. After four weeks of treatment, 67 percent of the participants experienced a positive improvement.

Basic Formula for Depression

St. John's wort 2 parts
Oats 1 part
Lavender 1 part
Mugwort 1 part
Take 1 tsp. of tincture 3 times a day for at least 1 month.

Other lifestyle issues must also be addressed in the treatment of depression. From green salads to relaxation, from spinal adjustments to listening to music, the list is endless. Exercise is especially important. The *Textbook of Natural Medicine* by Joseph Pizzorno, and Michael Murray N.D. suggests the following nutritional supplements:

- B vitamin complex, 50–150 mg daily
- Vitamin C, 1 gram 3 times daily
- Folic acid, 400 mcg daily
- Vitamin B_{12}, 250 mcg daily
- Magnesium, 500 mg daily

Insomnia

Insomnia is defined as an individual's perception that his or her sleep is inadequate or abnormal. The signs of insomnia include difficulty in falling asleep, frequent awakenings from sleep, a short sleep time, and nonrestorative sleep. It is a problem of too little sleep; this makes a person irritable and tired. Typically seven to nine hours of good quality sleep are needed on a regular basis. Virtually everyone has experienced an occasional sleepless night that leaves him incapacitated to some degree the next day.

There are many herbs with reputations as effective sleep remedies; however the key to successful treatment of insomnia is to find the cause and to deal with it. This may be anything from deep grief to constipation. Psychological issues often need attention, and so do health problems causing pain or discomfort. Dietary indiscretions must be identified, as must environmental factors such as freeway noise or a snoring spouse.

Treatment should not depend upon substances alone, whether they are herbs or drugs. Here are some suggestions to help get a good night's rest:

- Sleep as much as you need to feel refreshed and healthy, but not more. Excessively long hours in bed seem to be related to shallow sleep.
- Try to get up at the same time each day, regardless of when you went to bed. This will help establish a sleep/wake rhythm.
- Exercise the same amount each day, preferably in late afternoon or early evening.
- Do some sort of physical activity each day to get rid of tension and tire your body, but nothing too strenuous just before bedtime.
- Make sure the bedroom is quiet. If you work night shifts and sleep during the day or live in a noisy area, consider ear plugs or an eye mask.
- Keep the temperature comfortable.
- Sleep on a quality mattress and foundation.
- Keep the bedroom dark.
- Don't lie in bed for hours staring at the walls. If you don't fall asleep after 15 or 20 minutes, it is best to get up and do something quiet until you become drowsy.

- Don't make your bed a place to watch TV, do paperwork or eat.
- A light snack may help; a heavy meal won't.
- Unless prescribed, don't nap during the day. For most people, this can throw off the sleep schedule by confusing the body.
- Natural sunlight during the day can be helpful for falling and staying asleep, so get outdoors even for a brief walk.
- Caffeine in the evening disturbs sleep, even if you're not aware of it.
- Alcohol causes fragmented sleep. Although it can be initially calming, liquor can interfere with the quality of your sleep.
- Chronic tobacco use disturbs sleep.
- Try not to rehash the day's problems or worry about tomorrow's.
- When you go to bed, relax your muscles, beginning with your feet and working your way up to your head.

Often the key to successful herbal treatments lies in focusing upon some part or function of the body that is experiencing problems. Hypnotics and nervines are best selected based on the role they play upon the system in question and not simply their strength as hypnotics. If an accompanying health problem affects a particular body system, then the hypnotic remedy can be selected as follows:

Circulatory system: **Motherwort, lime blossom, balm.**

Respiratory system: All of the hypnotics can help as antispasmodics in conditions such as asthma, if used at the right dose. **Wild lettuce** eases irritable coughs.

Digestive system: The relaxing nervines and carminatives are all important especially **chamomile, vervain, balm, hops** and **valerian.** The antispasmodic herbs will help with

intestinal colic, for example **hops, passionflower** and
valerian.

Urinary system: Hypnotics are important here when used
as muscle relaxants.

Reproductive system: Of special relevance would be **pulsatilla** and **black cohosh.**

Muscles and skeleton: All hypnotics will aid in reducing
muscle tension and even the pain associated with problems
in this system. They may be used internally or as lotions.
Especially important are **valerian** and **black cohosh.**

Skin: **Chamomile** and **cowslip** are healing, but otherwise
the value of hypnotics here is to ensure that the body has
a good recuperative rest each night.

   The appropriate sleeping remedy can also be selected
on the basis of their strength, bearing in mind the very
subjective nature and individual variability of human response to these herbs. We can roughly identify three
groupings:

Sleep Remedies

Mild: **Chamomile, balm, linden, red clover.**

Medium: **Pulsatilla, mugwort, motherwort, skullcap,
vervain.**

Strong: **Californian poppy, hops, wild lettuce, passionflower, Jamaican dogwood, valerian.**

   By selecting herbs that address specific health problems
that are contributing to the sleep difficulties, better results
are obtained rather than simply going for a strong
hypnotic.

Herbal combinations for insomnia

1. Equal parts

   - **Passionflower**
   - **Valerian**

   Take 1 tsp. of tincture 30 minutes before bedtime.

2. For insomnia associated with menopausal problems:

   Equal parts
   - **Passionflower**
   - **Valerian**
   - **Motherwort**

   Take 1 tsp. of tincture 30 minutes before bedtime in addition
   to appropriate daytime treatments.

3. For insomnia associated with indigestion:

   Equal parts
   - **Mugwort**
   - **Balm**
   - **Passionflower**
   - **Valerian**

   Take 1½ tsp. of tincture 30 minutes before bedtime in addition
   to appropriate daytime treatments. An infusion of **chamomile,
   linden** or **balm** tea at night would also be helpful.

4. For insomnia associated with depression:

   Equal parts of
   - **St. John's wort**
   - **Mugwort**
   - **Passionflower**
   - **Valerian**

   Take 1½ tsp. of tincture 30 minutes before bedtime in addition
   to appropriate daytime treatments.

Avoid the use of **hops** in depression.

Indigestion

Digestive system symptoms can be an unpleasant way
for the stress response to manifest.

Every herbalist and every culture have their favorite
remedies for indigestion. European specifics include **gentian, peppermint, chamomile, balm, hops** and **valerian.**
Often a tea made from a single fresh remedy is best. This

should be an herb with a taste and aroma. Ideally it should be a plant you could easily cultivate, thus providing a steady supply of fresh leaf.

These simple teas can be augmented by using the following combination of tinctures to aid the digestive system in general:

Indigestion Tincture

Equal parts
- **Gentian**
- **Valerian**
- **Chamomile**
- **Peppermint**

Take ½ tsp 10 minutes before eating.

Hypertension

There are over 35 million hypertensives in the U.S., with twice as many African-Americans as Caucasians. The reasons for this are not known. Although hypertension is a common problem in our culture, it is rare in cultures that are relatively untouched by the Western lifestyle. Stress plays a major role in causing and maintaining hypertension. Dietary, psychological and social factors must all be addressed for any real change to occur.

A number of herbs are specific for hypertension, usually working because of their impact on one or another of the processes involved in the condition's development The most important plant remedy within Western medicine is **hawthorn**, probably followed by **linden. Garlic** is also effective for lowering high blood pressure and should be used in cooking and as a dietary supplement.

Hypertension Formula

- **Hawthorn** 2 parts
- **Linden** 1 part
- **Yarrow** 1 part
- **Crampbark** 1 part
- **Valerian** 1 part

Take 1 tsp. of tincture 3 times a day.

Other plants might also be included depending upon the specific symptoms. Here is a possible mixture for hypertension where stress is a major factor.

- **Hawthorn** 2 parts
- **Linden** 1 part
- **Yarrow** 1 part
- **Siberian ginseng** 1 part
- **Skullcap** 1 part
- **Crampbark** 1 part
- **Valerian** 1 part

Take 1 tsp. of tincture 3 times a day.

Premenstrual Syndrome (PMS)

This describes a broad range of symptoms that occur cyclically and which are severe enough to disturb a woman's life patterns or cause her to seek help from a health practitioner. Most women experience some body change cyclically during the menstruating years corresponding to the pattern of cycling hormones.

From my clinical experience I would suggest **skullcap** as ideally suited for relief of the psychological symptoms though various other remedies may act as well for specific women, so generalizations are problematic. Longer term hormonally focused herbal treatments are very effective but beyond the scope of this book.

The usual dosage of **skullcap** would be 1 heaped teaspoon of dried herb to 1 cup of boiling water taken three times a day or ¼ teaspoon of the tincture. This dosage may be increased until the desired relief is experienced. The dosage regime may be altered as necessary, varying time of day and quantity to suit individual needs. For example, one may take the whole dose first thing in the morning, or smaller amounts at frequent intervals throughout the day. The woman's experience is the guiding principle here.

Stress and Children

With its focus on preventive medicine, holistic approaches to health can be helpful in many of the common problems of childhood. If conditions are brought under control during childhood, they can often be avoided entirely in adult life. Children have special needs and special plants address these needs, but the most important consideration is the importance of tender loving care. Children respond to love and caring in wonderful ways. So do adults, if they give themselves the chance!

Children are susceptible to a variety of stresses, usually characterized by the feeling of being overwhelmed or threatened by more pressures and demands than they can handle. What constitutes a source of stress varies among children. One child may be stressed by changes in his daily routine, moving to a new home, or by the birth of a sibling. These same events may strike another child as novel, enjoyable and she may even thrive on such stimulation. Children also differ in their resilience and in how long it takes them to bounce back after stressful life events.

Coping usually requires thinking through the alternatives at hand and trying to make the best of stressful circumstances. However, a preschooler's capacity to analyze and formulate strategic plans is very limited. Getting help is therefore highly dependent upon an adult recognizing warning signs in youngsters struggling with stress. Once the problem is identified, the adult can help by listening to the child's expressions concerning stressful events and situations and offering understanding, support, reassurance and abundant affection, holding and cuddling. Coping with stress is easier when the child has a sense of self-esteem, which parents can and should encourage, and when they have good verbal and problem-solving skills. Children also learn coping strategies by observing others around them. When adults exhibit calmness in the face of emergencies or other difficulties, children learn from this example and are less likely to pick up fears and more likely to be able to cope with their own moments of difficulty.

A few of the many nervine remedies offered by nature are especially appropriate for problems of stress in children.

Procedure: Make an infusion using one-half to one teaspoon of the mixed herbs to one cup boiling water. Sweeten with honey. The dosage is one cup three times a day. Alternatively, add 10 drops of the mixed herbs in tincture form to a cup of juice.

Nervine Tonics
- Oats
- St. John's wort
- Skullcap

Nervine Relaxants
- Hyssop
- Lavender
- Chamomile
- Balm
- Linden
- Red clover

Hypnotics
- California poppy
- Chamomile

Here is a formulation created by Maribeth Riggs for overexcitability, anxiousness or mild insomnia.

INFANT'S CALMING HERBAL BATH

    1 qt. water
    1 oz. dried lavender buds
    1 oz. dried camomile flowers

1. Bring the water to a boil in a covered pot.
2. Remove the pot from the heat and add the herbs, being sure to cover the pot again. Let the herbs steep in the hot water for 20 minutes.
3. Strain and discard them. The bath tea is dark yellow and smells pleasantly of lavender.
4. Pour the tea into an infant bathtub and add enough warm water to fill it. The herbal bath should be as hot as a normal bath for the infant.

Application: Make sure the room is warm before the bath. Place the infant in the bathwater and hold him or her reassuringly, humming and crooning all the while. Soak the infant in the bath for at least 10 minutes. Do not try to wash the infant during an herbal bath. Gently pour the water over the belly and legs and just let the infant play and splash. Use this bath as often as necessary to reassure and calm an upset, colicky infant.

Hyperactivity. This is a thorny issue that raises a plethora of questions. There is no doubt that extreme hyperactivity occurs and can be related to dietary factors. This having been said, there is an unfortunate tendency for children to be labeled "hyperactive" simply because the teacher or parents do not have the patience for a very active, perceptive, inquisitive or creative child.

The Merck manual points out, quite rightly, that "claims that a child is hyperactive often reflect the tolerance level of the annoyed person." Since when has not fitting into the normal mold been a disease? The use of psychopharmaceuticals to control these children sounds a little bit like Soviet psychiatrists giving major tranquilizers to dissidents because they must (obviously) be insane to question the status quo. Rather than sedating our children so they can deal with their world, why not change the nature of schooling so it is more challenging and exciting?

Where the child is experiencing a real problem there may be some help that can be provided herbally, provided that two areas are first addressed:

- Psychological factors.
- Food irritants. There is increasing evidence that food or chemical irritants play a significant role in hyperactivity. They may be pollutants (such as heavy metals) or artificial food additives (such as colorings or flavors).

For details and support with these two areas contact The Feingold Association, 56 Winston Drive, Smithtown, NY 11787. (516) 543-4658.

Herbs to consider in supporting a broad treatment plan that also includes dietary psychological aspects, might be:

- Red clover
- Linden blossom
- Chamomile
- Milk thistle

These herbs can help with stress and exhaustion in the parents! For preparation and dosage instructions, see the procedure on pages 71–73.

THE HERBAL

This section contains brief descriptions of the uses and dosage for the herbs described in the book. The major herbs for stress, **chamomile** and **valerian**, are discussed first. The rest follow in alphabetical order.

Chamomile

Matricaria recutita

Part used: Flowering tops.
Actions: Nervine, anti-spasmodic, carminative, anti-inflammatory, antimicrobial, bitter, vulnerary.
Indications: A comprehensive list of chamomile's medical uses would be very long indeed. Included would be insomnia, anxiety, menopausal depression, loss of appetite, dyspepsia, diarrhea, colic, aches and pains of flu, migraine, neuralgia, teething, vertigo, motion sickness, conjunctivitis, inflamed skin, urticaria and on and on. This may seem too good to be true, but it reflects this herb's wide range of actions in the body.

Chamomile is probably the most widely used relaxing nervine herb in the Western world. It relaxes and tones the nervous system, and is especially valuable where anxiety and tension produce digestive symptoms such as gas, colic pains or even ulcers. The ability to focus on physical symptoms as well as underlying psychological tension is one of the great benefits of herbal remedies in stress and anxiety problems. Safe in all types of stress and anxiety-related problems, it makes a wonderful late-night tea to ensure restful sleep. It is also helpful with anxious children or teething infants, where it can be used as an addition to the bath.

As an antispasmodic herb, chamomile works on the peripheral nerves and muscles, thus indirectly relaxing the whole body. When the physical body is at ease, ease in the mind and heart follows. It can prevent or lessen cramps in the muscles, such as in the legs or abdomen. As the essential oil added to a bath, chamomile relaxes the body after a hard day while easing the cares and weight of a troubled heart and mind.

Being rich in essential oils, chamomile also acts on the digestive system, promoting proper function. This usually involves soothing the walls of the intestines, easing griping pains and helping with the removal of gas. It is an effective anti-inflammatory remedy internally for the digestive and respiratory systems as well as externally on the skin. A cup of hot chamomile tea is a simple, effective way of relieving indigestion, calming inflammations such as gastritis and helping prevent ulcer formation. Using the essential oil as a steam inhalation will allow the same oils to reach inflamed mucus membranes in the sinuses and lungs.

Chamomile is a mild antimicrobial, helping the body to destroy or resist pathogenic microorganisms. Azulene, one of the components of the essential oil, is bactericidal to *staphylococcus* and *streptoccus* infections. The oil from 0.10 g of flowers is enough to destroy three times the amount of staphylococcal toxins in two hours.

As an anticatarrhal, chamomile helps the body remove excess mucus buildup in the sinus area. It may be used in head colds and allergy reactions such as hay fever. Mucous is not a problem in itself, it is an essential body product. However, when too much is produced it is usually in response to an infection, helping the body remove the bacteria or excess carbohydrate from the body.

A review of recent scientific literature shows how much interest this venerable folk remedy is still receiving. Most of the clinical therapeutic research comes from Europe, reflecting the respect chamomile receives in the medical community there. Anti-inflammatory effects have been the main focus of research, being the official criteria for its inclusion in the Pharmacopoeia. These properties explain the herb's value in a wide range of digestive and intestinal problems. Taken by mouth or used as an enema chamomile is particularly helpful in colitis and irritable bowel syndrome. A fascinating recent German study demonstrated the efficacy of chamomile on the healing of wounds caused by tattooing. A common problem with tattoos is a "weeping" wound where the skin has been abraded. The healing and drying process was compared between patients who were treated with chamomile and a similar group that was not. The decrease of the weeping wound area as well as the speed of drying was dramatically improved using chamomile.

Clinical and laboratory research demonstrates statistically what the herbalist knows experientially, that chamomile will reduce inflammation, colic pain and protect against ulcer formation in the whole of the digestive tract. **Dosage:** The herb may be used in all the ways plants can be prepared as medicines. Used fresh or dried it can be infused to make a tea. A tincture is an excellent way of ensuring that all the plant's components are extracted and available for the body. In aromatherapy the essential oil of chamomile is a valued preparation. *Infusion:* 2-3 teaspoonfuls infused in 1 cup boiling water for 10 minutes. Drink 1 cup 3-4 times a day. *Tincture:* ¼-¾ tsp 3 times a day.

Valerian   *Valeriana officinalis*

Part used: Rhizome, stolons and roots.
Actions: Nervine, hypnotic, antispasmodic, carminative, hypotensive.
Indications: Valerian has a wide range of specific uses, but its main indications are anxiety, nervous sleeplessness, and the bodily symptoms of tension such as muscle cramping or indigestion. It may be used safely in situations

where tension and anxiety are causing problems. This may manifest in purely psychological and behavioral ways or also with physical symptoms. Valerian will help in most cases. For some people it can be an effective mild pain reliever.

As one of the best gentle and harmless herbal sleeping remedies, valerian enhances the natural body process of slipping into sleep and making the stress of the day recede. For people who do not need as much sleep as they once did, it also eases lying awake in bed, ensuring that it becomes a restful and relaxing experience. This can often be as revivifying as sleep itself, and indeed all that is necessary in many cases. The true nature of sleep still remains a mystery. Everybody goes through stages of REM (rapid eye movement) sleep, a stage where dreaming is associated with minor involuntary muscle jerks and rapid eye movements, indicating that active processes are occurring in the brain. It is important not to suppress the dreaming during this stage. Emotional experiences are processed by the mind in those dreams, and much arising from both the unconscious and daily life is balanced and harmonized. While sleeping pills have a marked impact on REM sleep, supressing dreaming, valerian does not interfere with this process because it is not powerful enough.

The research into valerian confirms the traditional experience of the herbalist. In one study valerian produced a significant decrease in subjectively evaluated sleep scores and an improvement in sleep quality. Improvement was most notable among those who considered themselves poor or irregular sleepers and smokers. Dream recall was relatively unaffected by valerian. When the effect of valerian root on sleep was studied in healthy young people, it reduced perceived sleep latency and the wake time after sleep onset. In other words the subjects experienced an easier and quicker descent into sleep. A combination of valerian and hops was given to people whose sleep was disturbed by heavy traffic noise. Giving the herbs well before retiring reduced the noise-induced disturbance of a number of sleep-stage patterns.

Much research has centered on valerian's effects upon smooth muscle, demonstrating that it is a powerful and safe muscle relaxant. It can be safely used in muscle cramping, uterine cramps and intestinal colic. Its sedative and antispasmodic action can be partially ascribed to the *valepotriates* and to a lesser extent to the *sesquiterpene* constituents of the volatile oils. Among other effects, valerian decreases both spontaneous and caffeine-stimulated muscular activity, significantly reduces aggressiveness in animals and decreases a number of measurable processes in the brain.

Italian researchers compared the relaxing properties of valerian with a number of other plants on the muscles of the digestive tract. Hawthorn and valerian were the most effective, followed by passionflower and chamomile. Especially interesting was the finding that combining all the herbs acted in a synergistic way, yielding relaxation at low dosage levels.

Valerian is used worldwide as a relaxing remedy in hypertension and stress-related heart problems. There is an effect here beyond simple nerve relaxation, as it contains alkaloids that are mild hypotensives. Such use is recognized by the World Health Organization, which promotes research and development of traditional medicine, understanding the importance of using whole plants and going beyond the test tube for meaningful results. In WHO-sponsored studies in Bulgaria, traditional herbs known for their healing effect in cardiovascular problems were studied and the results were impressive. Valerian is one such herb whose use was validated. Others were garlic, geranium, European Mistletoe, olive and hawthorn.

Dosage: To be effective valerian has to be used in sufficiently high dosage. The tincture is the most widely used preparation and is always useful, provided that the single dose is not counted in drops, but that ½-1 teaspoonful is given, and indeed sometimes 2 tsp. at one time. It is almost pointless to give 10 or 20 drops of valerian tincture. Overdosage is highly unlikely, even with much larger doses. For situations of extreme stress where a sedative or muscle relaxant effect is needed fast, the single dose of 1 teaspoonful may be repeated 2 or 3 times at short intervals.

The dried herb is prepared as an infusion to ensure no loss of the volatile oils. Use 1 to 2 teaspoons of the dried herb for each cup of tea prepared. With these doses expect a good relaxing, antispasmodic and sleep-inducing effect, and above all rapid sedation in states of excitement. A cold infusion may be used: a cup of cold water is poured over one to two teaspoons of valerian root and left to stand for 8-10 hours. A nighttime dose is thus set up in the morning, and a dose for the mornings is prepared at night.

Ashwagandha *Withania somnifera*

Part used: Root.

Actions: Adaptogen, sedative.

Indications: Ashwagandha is an herb from India used for the treatment of debility, impotence and premature aging. Modern research has stressed its antitumour and adaptogenic actions, reinforcing its comparison with ginseng. However, ashwagandha occupies an important place in the herbal *materia medica,* because while it is not as potent as panax ginseng, it lacks the stimulating effects of the latter. In fact it has a mild sedative action as indicated by its specific name *somnifera.* This makes it ideally suited to the treatment of overactive but debilitated people. Its indications include debility and nervous exhaustion especially due to stress, convalescence after acute illness or extreme stress and chronic inflammatory diseases especially of connective tissue. It is ideally suited as a general tonic for disease prevention and for those under stress.

Preparation and dosage: *Infusion:* put ½ teaspoonful of

the root in 1 cup of water, bring to the boil and simmer
gently for 10 minutes. Drink 1 cup, 3 times a day.
Tincture: take ¼-½ tsp. of the tincture 3 times a day.

Balm   *Melissa officinalis*

Part used: Dried aerial parts, or fresh in season.
Actions: Carminative, nervine, antispasmodic, diaphoretic, antimicrobial.
Indications: Balm is a relaxing, carminative herb that relieves spasms in the digestive tract and is often used in
flatulent dyspepsia. It is especially helpful where there is
dyspepsia associated with anxiety or depression, as the gently
sedative oils relieve tension and anxiety reactions. It may also
be used in migraine that is associated with tension, neuralgia,
anxiety-induced palpitations or insomnia. Extracts have antiviral properties and a lotion-based extract may be used for
skin lesions of *herpes simplex*, the antiviral activity having
been confirmed in both laboratory and clinical trials.
Preparations and dosage: *Infusion:* pour 1 cup of boiling
water onto 1-2 teaspoonfuls of the dried herb or 4-6 fresh
leaves and leave to infuse for 10-15 minutes, well covered.
Take 1 cup of this tea in the morning and the evening, or
when needed.
Tincture: take ¼-½ tsp. of the tincture 3 times a day.

Black Cohosh   *Cimicifuga racemosa*

Part used: Root and rhizome; dried, not fresh.
Actions: Emmenagogue, antispasmodic, nervine,
hypotensive.
Indications: Black cohosh offers a valuable combination
of actions that makes it uniquely useful in painful cramping conditions of the female reproductive system. It may
be used in cases of painful or delayed menstruation and
ovarian cramps. It is also active in the treatment of rheumatic, muscular and neurological pain. It is helpful in sci-

atica and neuralgia. As a relaxing nervine it may be used
in many situations where such an agent is needed. It has
been found beneficial in cases of tinnitus.

Preparations and dosage: *Decoction:* pour 1 cup of water
onto ½-1 teaspoonful of the dried root and bring to boil.
Let it simmer for 10-15 minutes. Drink 1 cup 3 times
a day.
Tincture: take ¼-½ tsp. of the tincture 3 times a day.

Black Haw   *Viburnum prunifolium*

Part used: Dried bark of root, stem or trunk.
Actions: Antispasmodic, hypotensive, astringent.
Indications: Black Haw has very similar use to crampbark, to which it is closely related. It is an effective relaxant of the uterus and is used for dysmenorrhea and false
labor pains as well as in threatened miscarriage. Its relaxant and sedative actions might explain its power in reducing blood pressure in hypertension, which happens through
a relaxation of the peripheral blood vessels. It may be used
as an antispasmodic in the treatment of asthma.
Preparations and dosage: *Decoction:* put 2 teaspoonfuls
of the dried bark in 1 cup of water, bring to the boil and
simmer for 10 minutes. Drink 1 cup 3 times a day.
Tincture: take—½-1 tsp. of the tincture 3 times a day.

Californian Poppy

Eschscholzia californica

Part used: Dried aerial parts.
Actions: Nervine, hypnotic, antispasmodic, anodyne.
Indications: A good general relaxing herb, it has been
used as a sedative and hypnotic for children when there
is overexcitability and sleeplessness. It can be used when-
ever an antispasmodic remedy is required.
Preparations and dosage: *Infusion:* pour a cup of boiling

water onto 1-2 teaspoonfuls of the dried herb and leave
to infuse for 10 minutes. Drink a cup at night to promote
restful sleep.

Tincture: take ¼-¾ tsp. of the tincture at night.

Celery Seed   *Apium graveolens*

Part used: Dried ripe fruits.
Actions: Antirheumatic, anti-inflammatory, diuretic, carminative, antispasmodic, nervine.
Indications: Celery seeds find their main use as a compo-
nent in the treatment of rheumatism, arthritis and gout.
They are especially useful in rheumatoid arthritis where
there is associated anxiety and mild depression. Their diuretic action is obviously involved in rheumatic conditions,
but they are also used as a urinary antiseptic, largely because of the volatile oil *apiol.*
Preparations and dosage: *Infusion:* pour 1 cup of boiling
water onto 1-2 teaspoonfuls of freshly crushed seeds.
Leave to infuse for 10-15 minutes. Drink 1 cup 3 times
a day.
Tincture: ½-¾ tsp. 3 times a day.

Crampbark   *Viburnum opulus*

Part used: Dried bark.
Actions: Antispasmodic, anti-inflammatory, nervine, hypotensive, astringent.
Indications: Crampbark shows by its name the richly de-
served reputation it has as a relaxer of muscular tension
and spasm. It has two main areas of use, in muscular
cramps and in **ovarian** and **uterine** muscle problems.
Crampbark will relax the uterus and so relieve painful
cramps associated with menstrual periods. In a similar way
it may be used to protect from threatened miscarriage. Its
astringent action gives it a role in the treatment of excessive menstrual blood loss, especially when associated
with menopause.

Preparations and dosage: *Decoction:* put 2 teaspoonfuls of the dried bark into a cup of water and bring to the boil. Simmer gently for 10-15 minutes. Drink hot 3 times a day. *Tincture:* take ¾-1½ tsp of the tincture 3 times a day.

Damiana   *Turnera diffusa*

Part used: Dried leaves and stems.
Actions: Nerve tonic, antidepressant, urinary antiseptic, laxative.
Indications: Damiana is a tonic strengthening remedy for the nervous system in debilitated people. It has an ancient reputation as an aphrodisiac. While this may or may not be true, it has a definite tonic action on the central nervous and endocrine systems. As a useful antidepressant, damiana is considered to be a specific in cases of anxiety and depression where there is a sexual factor. It may be used to strengthen the male sexual system.
Preparations and dosage: *Infusion:* pour 1 cup of boiling water onto 1 teaspoonful of the dried leaves and let infuse for 10-15 minutes. Drink 1 cup 3 times a day.
Tincture: take ¼-½ tsp. ml of the tincture 3 times a day.

Ginkgo   *Gingko biloba*

Part used: Leaves.
Actions: Anti-inflammatory, vasodilator.
Indications: Recent research has confirmed gingko's profound activity on brain function and cerebral circulation, thereby proving effective in a range of vascular disorders, especially those due to restricted cerebral blood flow and milder problems of normal aging such as weak memory, poor concentration and depression. Gingko has been suggested for the following conditions:

- Vertigo.
- Tinnitus.
- Inner ear disturbances including partial deafness.

- Impairment of memory and ability to concentrate.
- Diminished intellectual capacity and alertness as a result of insufficient circulation.
- Anxiety, depression, neurological disorders.
- Dementia, Alzeimer's disease.
- Complications of stroke and skull injuries.
- Diminished sight and hearing ability due to vascular insufficiency.
- Intermittent claudication as a result of arterial obstruction.
- A sensitivity to cold and pallor in the toes due to peripheral circulatory insufficiency.
- Raynaud's disease.
- Cerebral, vascular and nutritional insufficiency.
- Hormonal and neural-based disorders as well as angiopathic trophic disorders.
- Arterial circulatory disturbances due to aging, diabetes and nicotine abuse.
- Sclerosis of cerebral arteries with and without mental manifestations.
- Arteriosclerotic angiopathy of lower limbs.
- Diabetic tissue damage with danger of gangrene.
- Chronic arterial obliteration.
- Circulatory disorders of the skin.

Preparations and dosage: Gingko is becoming available in a number of different forms. The daily dose used in most studies was 27 mg of gingko flavone glycosides which corresponds to 6 to 12 g of leaf, depending on the quality of the leaf. Tablets or tinctures are usually standardized to contain 22.5 flavone glycosides and hence is highly concentrated compared to the original leaf. In the case of standardized liquid forms the dose is usually ¼ tsp. 3 times a day.

Ginseng, Korean and American

Panax spp.

Habitat: *Panax ginseng* is native to China and cultivated extensively in China, Korea, Japan and Russia. *Panax quinquefolia* is native to North America.

Part used: Root.

Actions: Adaptogen, tonic, stimulant, hypoglycemic.

Indications: Ginseng has an ancient history and as such has accumulated much folklore about its actions and uses. The genus name *panax* derives from the latin panacea meaning "cure all." Many of the claims that surround it are, unfortunately, exaggerated, but it is clear that this is an important remedy. A powerful adaptogen, ginseng has a wide range of possible therapeutic uses, the best being with weakness or old age, where the adaptogenic and stimulating properties can be profoundly useful. It should not be used indiscriminately as the stimulating properties can be contraindicated in some pathologies; for example, Chinese herbalism warns against using ginseng in acute inflammatory disease and bronchitis.

Preparations and dosage: *Decoction:* put ½-1 teaspoonful of the root in 1 cup of water, bring to the boil and simmer gently for 10 minutes. Drink 1 cup 3 times a day. *Tincture:* take ¼ -½ tsp. of the tincture 3 times a day for up to 3 months.

Hops

Humulus lupulus

Part used: Flowers.

Actions: Sedative, hypnotic, antimicrobial, antispasmodic, astringent.

Indications: Hops is a remedy that has a marked relaxing effect upon the central nervous system. It is used extensively for the treatment of insomnia. It will ease tension and anxiety and may be used where this tension leads to restlessness, headache and possibly indigestion. As an astringent with these relaxing properties it can be used in conditions such as mucous colitis. It should, however, be avoided where there is a marked degree of depression as this may be accentuated. Externally the antiseptic action is utilized for the treatment of ulcers.

CAUTION: Do not use when depression is present.

Preparations and dosage: *Infusion:* pour 1 cup of boiling water onto 1 teaspoonful of the dried flowers and let infuse for 10-15 minutes. Drink at night to induce sleep. This dose may be strengthened if needed.

Tincture: take ¼-½ tsp. of the tincture 3 times a day.

Hyssop   *Hyssopus officinalis*

Part used: Dried aerial parts.

Actions: Antispasmodic, expectorant, diaphoretic, nervine, anti-inflammatory, carminative.

Indications: Hyssop has an interesting range of uses which are largely attributable to the antispasmodic action of the volatile oil. It is used in coughs, bronchitis and chronic catarrh. Its diaphoretic properties explain its use in the common cold. As a nervine it may be used in anxiety states, hysteria and *petit mal* (a form of epilepsy).

Preparation and dosage: *Infusion:* pour 1 cup of boiling water onto 1-2 teaspoonfuls of the dried herb and leave to infuse for 10-15 minutes. Drink 1 cup 3 times a day.

Tincture: Take ¼-½ tsp. of the tincture 3 times a day.

Kava Kava   *Piper methysticum*

Part used: Rhizome

Actions: Relaxing nervine, hypnotic, anti-spasmodic, local anesthetic, anti-fungal.

Indications: Kava kava is a safe treatment for anxiety which at normal therapeutic doses does not dampen alertness or interact with mild alcohol consumption. It possesses a mild antidepressant activity making it suitable for the treatment of anxiety associated with minor forms of depression. Kava is an effective muscle relaxant, making it useful for the treatment of conditions associated with skeletal muscle spasm and tension, such as headaches due to neck tension. It is also a relevant hypnotic in cases of mild insomnia. The local anesthetic action on mucous membranes makes kava useful for pain control in oral conditions.

Preparations and dosage: *Decoction:* put 1-2 teaspoonfuls of the rhizome in a cup of water, bring to boiling and simmer gently for 10-15 minutes; drink as needed.

Tincture: take ½-1 tsp per day. Standardized preparations should supply 100 to 200 mg of kava lactones per day.

Kola
Cola vera

Part used: Seed kernel.

Actions: Stimulant to central nervous system, antidepressive, astringent, diuretic.

Indications: Kola has a marked stimulating effect on human consciousness. It can be used wherever there is a need for direct stimulation, which is less often than is usually thought. Through regaining proper health and therefore right functioning, the nervous system does not need such help. In the short term it may be used in nervous debility, in states of atony and weakness. It can act as a specific in nervous diarrhea. It will aid in states of depression and may in some people give rise to euphoric states. In some varieties of migraine it can help greatly. It can be viewed as specific in cases of depression associated with weakness and debility.

Preparations and dosage: *Decoction:* put 1-2 teaspoonfuls of the powdered nuts in 1 cup of water, bring to boiling and simmer gently for 10-15 minutes. Drink when needed.

Tincture: take ¼-½ tsp. of the tincture 3 times a day.

Lavender   *Lavandula officinalis*

Part used: Flowers.

Actions: Carminative, antispasmodic, antidepressant, emmenagogue, hypotensive.

Indications: This beautiful herb has many uses, culinary, cosmetic and medicinal. It is often an effective herb for headaches, especially when they are related to stress. Lavender can be quite effective in the clearing of depression, especially if used in conjunction with other remedies. As a gentle strengthening tonic of the nervous system it may be used in states of nervous debility and exhaustion. It can be used to soothe and promote natural sleep. Externally the oil may be used as a stimulating liniment to help ease the aches and pains of rheumatism.

Preparations and dosage: *Infusion:* to take internally, pour 1 cup of boiling water onto 1 teaspoonful of the dried herb and leave to infuse for 10 minutes. Drink 1 cup 3 times a day.

External use: the oil should not be taken internally but simply inhaling the aroma of lavender oil, rubbing a few drops onto the wrists or adding a few drops to your bath can be very relaxing.

Linden   *Tilia europea*

Part used: Dried flowers.

Actions: Nervine, antispasmodic, hypotensive, diaphoretic, diuretic, anti-inflammatory, astringent.

Indications: Linden is well known as a relaxing remedy for use in nervous tension. It has a reputation as a prophylactic against the development of arteriosclerosis and hypertension. It is considered to be a specific in the treatment of raised blood pressure associated with arteriosclerosis and nervous tension. Its relaxing action combined with a general effect upon the circulatory system give linden a role in the treat-

ment of some forms of migraine. The diaphoresis combined with the relaxation explain its value in feverish colds and flu.
Preparations and dosage: *Infusion:* pour 1 cup of boiling water onto 1 teaspoonful of the blossoms and leave to infuse for 10 minutes. Drink 1 cup 3 times a day. For a diaphoretic effect in fever, use 2-3 teaspoonfuls.
Tincture: take ¼-½ tsp. of the tincture 3 times a day.

Motherwort *Leonurus cardiaca*

Part used: Aerial parts.
Actions: Nervine, emmenagogue, antispasmodic, cardiac tonic, hypotensive.
Indications: The English and Latin names of this plant show its range of uses. *Motherwort* indicates its relevance to menstrual and uterine conditions while *cardiaca* indicates its use in heart and circulation treatments. It is valuable in the stimulation of delayed or suppressed menstruation, especially where there is anxiety or tension involved. It is a useful relaxing tonic for aiding in menopausal changes. It may be used to ease false labor pains. It is an excellent tonic for the heart, strengthening without straining. It is considered to be a specific in cases of tachycardia (heart palpitations), especially when brought about by anxiety and other such causes. It may be used in all heart conditions that are associated with anxiety and tension.
Preparations and dosage: *Infusion:* pour 1 cup of boiling water into 1-2 teaspoonfuls of the dried herb and leave to infuse for 10-15 minutes. Drink 1 cup 3 times a day.
Tincture: take ¼-¾ tsp. of the tincture 3 times a day.

Mugwort *Artemisia vulgaris*

Part used: Leaves or root.
Actions: Bitter tonic, nervine tonic, emmenagogue.
Indications: Mugwort can be used wherever a digestive stimulant is called for. It will aid the digestion through

the bitter stimulation of the juices while also providing a carminative oil. It has a mildly nervine action in aiding depression and easing **tension,** which appears to be due to the volatile oil. It is essential that the volatile oil is not lost in preparation. Mugwort may also be used as an emmenagogue in the aiding of normal menstrual flow.

Preparations and dosage: *Infusion:* pour 1 cup of boiling water onto 1-2 teaspoonfuls of the dried herb and leave to infuse for 10-15 minutes in a covered container. Drink 1 cup 3 times a day. Mugwort is used as a flavoring in a number of aperitif drinks such as vermouth, a pleasant way to take it!

Tincture: take ¼-½ tsp of the tincture 3 times a day.

Oats
Avena sativa

Part used: Seeds and whole plant.

Actions: Nervine tonic, antidepressant, nutritive, demulcent, vulnerary.

Indications: Oats is one of the best remedies for nourishing the nervous system, especially when under stress. It is considered a specific in cases of nervous debility and exhaustion when associated with depression. It may be used with most of the other nervines, both relaxant and stimulatory, to strengthen the whole of the nervous system. It is also used in general debility.

Preparations and dosage: *Infusion:* pour 1 cup of boiling water onto 1-3 teaspoonfuls of the dried oat straw and leave to infuse 10-15 minutes. Drink 1 cup 3 times a day.

Tincture: take ½-1 tsp. 3 times a day.

Bath: a soothing bath for use in neuralgia and irritated skin conditions can be made in the following ways. Boil 1 pound of shredded oat straw in 2 quarts of water for 30 minutes. Strain the liquid and add it to the bath water: Or cooked rolled oats may be put into a muslin bag which is put into the tub and used as a sponge to bathe with.

Pulsatilla *Anemone pulsatilla*

Part used: Aerial parts.
Actions: Nervine, antispasmodic, antibacterial.
Indications: Pulsatilla is an effective relaxing nervine for use in problems relating to nervous tension and spasm in the reproductive system. It may be used with safety in the relief of painful periods, ovarian pain and painful conditions of the testes. It may be used to reduce tension reactions and headaches associated with them. It will help insomnia and general overactivity. The antibacterial actions give this herb a role in treating infections that affect the skin, especially boils. It is similarly useful in the treatment of respiratory infections and asthma. The oil or tincture will ease earache.
Preparations and dosage: *Infusion:* pour 1 cup of boiling water over ½ teaspoonful of the dried herb and leave to infuse for 10-15 minutes. Drink 1 cup 3 times a day or when needed.
Tincture: ⅛-¼ tsp. 3 times a day.

Passionflower *Passiflora incarnata*

Part used: Leaves and whole plant.
Actions: Nervine, hypnotic, antispasmodic, anodyne, hypotensive.
Indications: Passionflower has a depressant effect on central nervous system activity and is hypotensive. It is used for its sedative and soothing properties, to lower blood pressure and for insomnia. The alkaloids and flavonoids have both been reported to have sedative activity in animals. Many of the flavonoids, such as *apigenin,* are well-known for pharmacological activity, particularly antispasmodic and anti-inflammatory activities. It is the herb of choice for treating intransigent insomnia. It aids the transition into a restful sleep without any narcotic hang-

over. It may be used wherever an anti-spasmodic is required, e.g. in Parkinson's disease, seizures and hysteria.
It can help in relieving nerve pain such as neuralgia and
the viral infection of nerves called shingles.

Preparations and dosage: *Infusion:* pour 1 cup of boiling
water onto 1-2 teaspoonfuls of the dried herb and let infuse
for 15 minutes. Drink 1 cup in the evening for sleeplessness and 1 cup 2 times a day for the easing of other
conditions. *Tincture:* take ¼-¾ tsp. of the tincture and use
in the same frequency as the infusion.

Red Clover   *Trifolium pratense*

Part used: Flower heads.
Actions: Alternative, expectorant, antispasmodic.
Indications: As a gentle, relaxing nervine, red clover has
a unique use as a safe and gentle sedative for hyperactive
children. It is also one of the most useful remedies for
children with skin problems. It may be used with complete
safety in any case of childhood eczema. It may also be of
value in other chronic skin conditions such as psoriasis.
Red clover can also be of value for adults. The expectorant
and antispasmodic action give this remedy a role in the
treatment of coughs and bronchitis, but especially in
whooping cough. As an alternative it is indicated in a wide
range of problems when approached in a holistic sense.
Preparations and dosage: *Infusion:* pour 1 cup of boiling
water onto 1-4 teaspoonfuls of the dried herb and leave
to infuse for 10-15 minutes. Drink 1 cup 3 times a day.
Tincture: take ½-¾ tsp. of the tincture 3 times a day.

Siberian Ginseng

Eleutherococcus senticosus

Part used: The root.
Actions: Adaptogen.
Indications: Siberian ginseng can be recommended as a

general tonic with a very wide range of clinical indications because of its nonspecific action. It is especially useful in conditions impacted by the stress response, including angina, hypertension, hypotension, various types of neuroses, chronic bronchitis and cancer and to treat the effects of prolonged stress or overwork such as exhaustion, irritability, insomnia and mild depression. Siberian ginseng can be used to assist recovery from acute or chronic diseases, trauma, surgery and other stressful episodes, as well as to counter the debilitating effects of chronic disease and treatments such as chemotherapy, radiation and surgery. It can be taken on a longterm basis to minimize the incidence of acute infections and to generally improve well-being.

Preparations and dosage: The standard dosage of the tincture, based upon clinical studies, ½-¾ tsp. 3 times a day. An equivalent dosage using a solid extract concentrated at a ratio of 20:1 would be 100-200 mg. The recommended regime is usually for a 6-week course followed by a 2-week break. This regime can be repeated for as long as is necessary.

Skullcap *Scutellaria laterifolia*

Part used: Aerial parts.

Actions: Nervine tonic, antispasmodic, hypotensive.

Indications: Skullcap is perhaps the most widely relevant nervine available to us in the *materia medica*. It relaxes states of nervous tension while at the same time renewing and revivifying the central nervous system. It has a specific use in the treatment of seizure and hysterical states as well as epilepsy. It may be used for exhaustion or depression. It can be used with complete safety in the easing of premenstrual syndrome.

Preparations and dosage: *Infusion:* pour 1 cup of boiling water onto 1-2 teaspoonfuls of the dried herb and leave to infuse for 10-15 minutes. Drink 1 cup 3 times a day or when needed. *Tincture:* take ½-¾ tsp. of the tincture 3 times a day.

St. John's Wort

Hypericum perforatum

Part used: Aerial parts.

Actions: Anti-inflammatory, antidepressant, astringent, vulnerary, nervine, antimicrobial.

Indications: Taken internally, St. John's wort has a sedative and mild pain-reducing effect, which gives it a place in the treatment of neuralgia, anxiety, tension and similar problems. It is especially helpful when there are menopausal changes triggering irritability and anxiety. It is increasingly recommended for the treatment of depression. The standardized extract is recognized by the German government as an effective treatment for depressive states, fear and nervous disturbances. In addition to neuralgic pain, it will ease fibrositis, sciatica and rheumatic pain. Externally it is a valuable healing and anti-inflammatory remedy. As a lotion it will speed the healing of wounds and bruises, varicose veins and mild burns. The oil is especially useful for the healing of sunburn.

Preparations and dosage: *Infusion:* pour 1 cup of boiling water onto 1-2 teaspoonfuls of the dried herb and leave to infuse for 10-15 minutes. Drink 1 cup 3 times a day. *Tincture:* take ¼-¾ tsp. of the tincture 3 times a day.

In the treatment of depression the recommended dose is 300 mg. 3 times daily of concentrated dry extract standardized to 0.3% hypericin.

Vervain

Verbena officinalis

Part used: Aerial parts.

Actions: Nervine tonic, sedative, antispasmodic, diaphoretic, hypotensive, galactagogue, hepatic.

Indications: Vervain is an herb that will strengthen the nervous system while relaxing any tension and stress. It can be used to ease depression and melancholia, especially when this follows illness such as influenza. Vervain may be used to help in seizure and hysteria. As a diaphoretic it can be used in the early stages of fevers. As a hepatic remedy it is helpful in jaundice and inflammation of the gallbladder. It may also be used as a mouthwash against caries and gum disease.

Preparations and dosage: *Infusion:* pour 1 cup of boiling water onto 1-4 teaspoonfuls of the dried herb and leave to infuse for 10-15 minutes. Drink 1 cup 3 times a day. *Tincture:* take ½-¾ tsp of the tincture 3 times a day.

Wild Cherry Bark *Prunus serotina*

Part used: Dried bark.

Actions: Antitussive, expectorant, astringent, nervine, antispasmodic.

Indications: While this herb is not a direct relaxing remedy, it may be used for easing stress- or tension-induced coughing or asthma. Due to its powerful sedative action on the cough reflex, wild cherry bark finds its main use in the treatment of irritating coughs and thus has a role in the treatment of bronchitis and whooping cough. It can be used with other herbs in the control of asthma. It must be remembered, however, that the inhibition of a cough does not equate with the healing of a chest infection, which will still need to be treated. It may also be used as a bitter where digestion is sluggish. The cold infusion of the bark may be helpful as a wash in cases of inflammation of the eyes.

Preparation and dosage: *Infusion:* pour 1 cup of boiling water onto 1-2 teaspoonfuls of the dried bark and leave to infuse for 10-15 minutes. Drink 1 cup 3 times a day. *Tincture:* take ¼-½ tsp. of the tincture 3 times a day.

Wild Lettuce   *Lactuca virosa*

Part used: Dried leaves.

Actions: Nervine, anodyne, hypnotic, antispasmodic.

Indications: The latex of the wild lettuce was at one time sold as "Lettuce Opium," naming the use of this herb quite well! It is a valuable remedy for use in insomnia, restlessness and excitability (especially in children) and other manifestations of an overactive nervous system. As an antispasmodic it can be used as part of a holistic treatment of whooping cough and dry irritated coughs in general. It will relieve colic pains in the intestines and uterus and so may be used in dysmenorrhea. It will also ease muscular pains related to rheumatism.

Preparations and dosage: *Infusion:* pour 1 cup of boiling water onto 1-2 teaspoonfuls of the leaves and let infuse for 10-15 minutes. Drink 1 cup 3 times a day.

Tincture: take ¼-½ tsp. of the tincture 3 times a day.

THE
PREPARATION
OF HERBAL
MEDICINES

From a therapeutic perspective, the basic way of using herbs is to take them internally since it is from within that healing takes place. The ways of preparing internal remedies are numerous, but with all of them it is essential to take care with the process to ensure you end up with what you want.

Teas

There are two ways to prepare teas: infusions and decoctions. There are some basic rules of thumb for choosing which method to use with what herb, but as with all generalizations, there are many exceptions.

Infusions are for nonwoody material such as leaves, flowers and some stems.

Decoctions are necessary if the herb contains any hard or woody material such as roots, barks or nuts. The denser the plant or the individual cell walls, the more energy is needed to extract cell content into the tea, thus explaining the value of decocting. An important exception would be a root rich in a volatile oil such as valerian root. The woodiness would suggest decocting, but if the roots are simmered the therapeutically important volatile oil would boil off.

To make an infusion:

- Take a china or glass teapot which has been warmed and put about 1 teaspoonful of the dried herb or herb mixture into it for each cup of tea.
- Pour 1 cup of boiling water in for each teaspoonful of herb that is already in the pot and then put the lid on. Leave to steep for 10 to 15 minutes. Infusions may be taken hot (which is normally best for a medicinal herb tea) cold or iced. They may be sweetened with liqorice root, honey or brown sugar. Any aromatic herb should be infused in a pot that has a tight-fitting lid to ensure that only a minimum of the volatile oil is lost through evaporation.

Herbal teabags can be made by filling little muslin bags with herbal mixtures, taking care to remember how many teaspoonfuls have been put into each bag! They can be used in the same way as ordinary tea bags. These teabags may be ordered from the suppliers listed in Appendix 3.

To make a decoction:

- Put 1 teaspoonful of dried herb or 3 teaspoonfuls of fresh material for each cup of water into a pot or saucepan. Dried herbs should be powdered or broken into small pieces, while fresh material should be cut into small pieces. If large quantities are made, use 1 ounce of dried herb for each pint of water. The container should be glass, ceramic or earthenware. If using metal it should be enameled.
- Add the appropriate amount of water to the herbs.
- Bring to a boil and simmer for the time given for the

mixture or specific herb, usually 10 to 15 minutes. If
the herb contains volatile oils, put a lid on.
- Strain the tea while still hot.

Tinctures

Alcohol preparations.   In general, alcohol is a
better solvent than water for plant constituents, so mixtures
of alcohol and water dissolve nearly all the relevant ingre-
dients of an herb and at the same time act as a preservative. Alcohol preparations are called tinctures, an
expression that is occasionally also used for preparations
based on glycerin or vinegar, as described below. The
method given here for the preparation of tinctures shows
a simple and general approach; when tinctures are prepared
professionally according to descriptions in a pharmacopoeia, specific water/alcohol proportions are used for each
herb, but for general use such details are unnecessary. For
home use it is best to take an alcohol of at least 30 percent
(60 proof) vodka for instance, as this is about the weakest
alcohol/water mixture with a long-term preservative action.

To make an alcoholic tincture

- Put 4 ounces of finely chopped or ground dried herb
  into a container that can be tightly closed. If fresh
  herbs are used, twice the amount should be taken.
- Pour 1 pint of 30 percent (60 proof) vodka on the
  herbs and close tightly.
- Keep the container in a warm place for 2 weeks and
  shake it well 2 times every day.
- After decanting the bulk of the liquid, pour the residue
  into a muslin cloth suspended in a bowl.
- Wring out all the liquid. The herbal residue makes
  excellent compost.
- Pour the tincture into a dark bottle. It should be kept
  well stoppered.

As tinctures are stronger than infusions or decoctions, the dosage to be taken is much smaller, depending on the herb. Tinctures may be used in a variety of ways. They can be taken straight, mixed with water or they can be added to a cup of hot water. If this is done, the alcohol will largely evaporate, leaving most of the extract in the water, possibly making the water cloudy, as resins and other constituents not soluble in water will precipitate. Some drops of the tincture can be added to a bath or footbath, used in a compress or mixed with oil and wax to make an ointment.

Another form of alcohol-based medicine are the liquid or fluid extracts. They are much more concentrated than tinctures with one part by volume of the fluid extract being equivalent to one part by weight of the herb.

Another way of making a kind of alcohol infusion is to infuse herbs in wine. Even though wine-based preparations do not have the shelf life of tinctures and are not as concentrated, they can be both pleasant to take and effective.

Glycerin-based tinctures. Tinctures based on glycerin have the advantage of being milder on the digestive tract and are best for children or for those sensitive to alcohol. However, they have the disadvantage of not dissolving resinous or oily materials very well. As a solvent glycerin is generally better than water but not as good as alcohol.

To make a glycerin tincture, make up 1 pint of a mixture consisting of 1 part glycerin and 1 part water, add 4 ounces of the dried ground herb and leave it in a well-stoppered container for 2 weeks, shaking it daily. After 2 weeks, strain and press or wring the residue as with alcoholic tinctures. For fresh herbs, due to their greater water content, put 8 oz. of herbs into a mixture of 75 percent glycerin/25 percent water.

Dry Preparations

Sometimes it is more appropriate to take herbs in a dry form, such as capsules or tablets. The advantage is that the taste of the herb can be avoided and the whole herb can be taken, including the woody material. There are, however, a number of drawbacks.

Because the dry herbs are unprocessed the plant constituents might not be readily available for easy absorption. During infusion, heat and water help to break down the walls of the plant cells and dissolve the constituents, which is not always guaranteed during the digestive process in the stomach and the small intestines. When the constituents are already dissolved in liquid form, they are available a lot faster and begin their action sooner.

Taking all this into account, there are still a number of ways to use herbs in dry form. The main thing to pay attention to is that the herbs be powdered as finely as possible. This guarantees that the cell walls are largely broken down and helps in the digestion and absorption of the herb. Unfortunately, the techniques used to grind the herb fine enough will also cause much heat generation through friction, which may lead to an unwanted change in the chemistry of the herb.

Capsules

The easiest way to use dry powdered herbs internally is to use gelatin capsules. Capsules not made of animal products are also produced. The size needed depends on the amount of herbs prescribed per dose, the density of the plant and on the volume of the material. A capsule size 00 holds about 0.5 grams (1/6 ounces) of finely powdered herb.

- Place the powdered herbs in a flat dish and take the halves of the capsule apart.

- Move the halves of the capsules through the powder, filling them in the process.
- Push the halves together.

Pills

There are a number of ways to make pills, depending on the degree of technical skill you possess. The simplest way to take an unpleasant remedy is to roll the powder into a small pill with fresh bread, which works most effectively with herbs such as goldenseal or cayenne.

- Grind herbs as fine as possible (a coffee grinder works well).
- Add a small amount of water and maple syrup to make a mud pie consistency.
- Knead in slippery elm powder to roll into small balls.

Baths

A pleasant way of absorbing herbal compounds through the skin is by bathing in a full body bath with 1 pint of an infusion or decoction added to the water. Any herb that can be taken internally can also be used in a bath. Herbs can, of course, also be used to give the bath a lovely fragrance.

For a bath that will bring out a deep and restful sleep, add an infusion of one of the hypnotic herbs to the bathwater. Bear in mind that although valerian and hops are very effective, their aroma is not pleasant.

- **Californian poppy**
- **Chamomile**
- **Hops**
- **Linden**
- **Motherwort**
- **Mugwort**
- **Passionflower**
- **Pulsatilla**
- **Skullcap**
- **Valerian**
- **Wild lettuce**

For children with sleep problems or when babies are teething, try adding the following herbs to the bath water:

- **Linden**
- **Chamomile**
- **Red clover**

Make an infusion as described above or place a handful of the herb in a muslin bag which is suspended from the hot water tap so the water flows through it. In this way a very fresh infusion can be made.

Essential Oils and Aromatherapy

Aromatherapy, a healing system based on the external application of herbs in the form of essential oils, has much to offer here. These oils can also be used in baths by putting a few drops of oil into the bathwater. The following brief summary of the oils comes from an excellent and comprehensive guide entitled *Aromatherapy* by Kathi Keville and Mindy Green.

Emotion	Essential oil
Anger	Basil, Chamomile, Cinnamon, Coriander, Frankincense, Geranium, Hyssop, Jasmine, Lavender, Melissa, Neroli, Pine, Rose, Rosewood, Ylang-ylang
Anxiety	Basil, Benzoin, Bergamot, Camphor, Cardamom, Chamomile, Cypress, Fennel, Frankincense, Geranium, Jasmine, Juniper, Lavender, Marjoram, Melissa, Nutmeg, Patchouli, Petitgrain, Peppermint, Pine, Rose, Rosemary, Rosewood, Sandalwood, Ylang-ylang
Apathy	Geranium, Jasmine, Neroli, Patchouli, Peppermint, Pine, Rose, Rosemary, Rosewood, Sage

Confusion	Basil, Camphor, Cardamom, Cedar, Cinnamon, Cypress, Frankincense, Helichrysum, Hyssop, Jasmine, Lavender, Lemon, Marjoram, Neroli, Patchouli, Peppermint, Sandalwood
Depression	Basil, Bergamot, Chamomile, Clary sage, Coriander, Frankincense, Geranium, Helichrysum, Lavender, Lemon, Neroli, Patchouli, Petitgrain, Peppermint, Pine, Rose, Rosewood, Sandalwood, Vetivert, Ylang-ylang
Fear	Basil, Chamomile, Coriander, Fennel, Hyssop, Jasmine, Melissa, Neroli, Orange, Rose, Thyme
Grief	Cypress, Hyssop, Jasmine, Marjoram, Rose, Rosemary, Sage
Hypersensitive	Cedar, Chamomile, Clary sage, Eucalyptus, Geranium, Hyssop, Juniper, Lavender, Marjoram, Myrrh, Neroli, Patchouli, Rose, Ylang-ylang
Impatience	Bergamot, Camphor, Chamomile, Fennel, Frankincense, Jasmine, Lavender, Marjoram, Myrrh, Rose
Instability	Anise, Benzoin, Bergamot, Camphor, Chamomile, Cypress, Geranium, Helichrysum, Hyssop, Lavender, Lemon, Marjoram, Myrrh, Rosemary, Sandalwood, Thyme
Insomnia	Bergamot, Chamomile, Cypress, Frankincense, Geranium, Jasmine, Lavender, Lemon, Marjoram, Melissa, Myrrh, Neroli, Nutmeg, Patchouli, Petitgrain, Rose, Sage, Sandalwood, Ylang-ylang
Melancholy	Benzoin, Frankincense, Lavender, Marjoram, Melissa, Peppermint, Rose, Rosemary, Rosewood, Sandalwood, Thyme
Panic/Shock	Bay, Camphor, Chamomile, Clary sage,

	Coriander, Eucalyptus, Jasmine, Lavender, Melissa, Orange, Patchouli, Petitgrain, Peppermint, Rosewood, Vetivert, Ylang-ylang
Stress	Anise, Basil, Bay, Bergamot, Cardamom, Chamomile, Clary Sage, Eucalyptus, Fennel, Frankincense, Helichrysum, Juniper, Lavender, Lemon, Marjoram, Neroli, Nutmeg, Orange, Peppermint, Rose, Rosewood, Sage, Sandalwood, Thyme, Ylang-ylang
Irritability	Cedar, Clary sage, Cinnamon, Cypress, Melissa, Neroli, Orange, Patchouli

There are a range of ways to use essential oils. The dilutions are for adults, so halve them for children, and use them at quarter strength for infants.

Massage oils. Always dilute oils before applying them to the skin. Use a carrier oil such as sweet almond oil, grapeseed oil, jojoba oil or any other pure, unblended vegetable oil. Do not use "baby oil," as this is a mineral oil and, unlike vegetable oils, will not be absorbed by the skin. 3-5 drops of essential oil to 2 tsp. of a carrier oil is usually appropriate.

Baths. Add up to 5 drops of pure essential oil to a bath full of warm water. Float the oil on the surface and stir with your hand before relaxing in the bath for 10-15 minutes. For a hand or foot soak use 2-3 drops in a bowl of warm water.

Inhalation. Add 2 drops of essential oil to a bowl of hot water, cover your head with a towel and inhale the fragrant steam.

Herbalists Kathi Keville and Mindy Green also suggest these formulas which can be used as a massage or bath oil.

Relaxing/antidepressant Formula

- 3 drops lavender
- 3 drops neroli
- 2 drops marjoram
- 2 drops ylang-ylang
- 1 drop chamomile
- 2 drops clary sage
- 1 ounce carrier oil

Adrenal Support Formula

- 4 drops pine
- 4 drops spruce
- 2 drops lavender
- 1 ounce carrier oil

This blend can be used in the bath or as a massage oil. For extra stimulation add 2 drops rosemary.

APPENDIX

Actions of Herbs

Adaptogens increase resistance and resilience to stress, enabling the body to avoid collapse by adapting to the problem. Adaptogens appear to work through support of the adrenal glands.

Alteratives gradually restore proper functioning of the body, increasing health and vitality. Some alternatives support natural waste elimination via the kidneys, liver, lungs or skin. Others stimulate digestive function or are antimicrobial.

Anti-catarrhals help the body remove excess mucous, whether in the sinus area or other parts of the body. Catarrh is not of itself a problem, but when too much is produced it is usually in response to an infection or excess carbohydrate in the body.

Anti-inflammatories soothe inflammations or reduce the inflammation of the tissue directly. They work in a number of different ways, but rarely inhibit the natural inflammatory reaction as such; rather they support and encourage the work the body is undertaking.

Antimicrobials help the body destroy or resist pathogenic microorganisms. They help the body strengthen its own resistance to infective organisms and throw off the illness. While some contain chemicals which are antiseptic or specific poisons to certain organisms, in general they aid the body's natural immunity.

Antispasmodics ease cramps in muscles. They alleviate

muscular tension and, as many are also nervines, ease psychological tension as well. There are antispasmodics that reduce muscle spasms throughout the body and also those that work on specific organs or systems.

Astringents have a binding action on mucous membranes, skin and other tissue, due to chemicals called *tannins*. They have the effect of precipitating protein molecules thus reducing irritation and inflammation, creating a barrier against infection that is helpful in wounds and burns.

Bitters are herbs with a bitter taste, with a special role in preventative medicine. The taste triggers a sensory response in the central nervous system. A message goes to the gut releasing digestive hormones leading to a range of actions including the stimulation of appetite as well as flow of digestive juices; an aid to the liver's detoxification work and an increased bile flow. Bitters also stimulate gut self-repair mechanisms.

Cardiac remedies have a beneficial action on the heart. Some of the remedies in this group are powerful cardioactive agents such as foxglove, whereas others are gentler, safer herbs such as hawthorn and motherwort.

Carminatives are rich in aromatic volatile oils that stimulate the digestive system to work properly and with ease, soothing the gut wall, reducing any inflammation that might be present, easing gripping pains and helping to remove gas from the digestive tract.

Demulcents are rich in mucilage that soothes and protects irritated or inflamed tissue. They reduce irritation down the whole length of the bowel, reduce sensitivity to potentially corrosive gastric acids, help to prevent diarrhea and reduce the muscle spasms which cause colic. They also ease coughing by soothing bronchial tension and relax painful spasm in the bladder.

Diaphoretics promote perspiration, helping the skin eliminate waste from the body, thus helping the body ensure a clean and harmonious inner environment. Some produce observable sweat, while others aid normal background perspiration. They often promote dilation of surface capillaries, so helping improve poor circulation. They support the work of the kidneys by increasing cleansing through the skin.

Diuretics increase the production and elimination of urine. In herbal medicine, with its ancient traditions, the term is often applied to herbs that have a beneficial action on the urinary system. They help the body eliminate waste and support the whole process of inner cleansing.

Emmenagogues stimulate menstrual flow and activity. In most herbals, however, the term is used in the wider sense of a remedy that normalizes and tones the female reproductive system.

Expectorants are herbs that stimulate removal of mucous from the lungs, and they are a tonic for the entire respiratory system. Stimulating expectorants irritate the bronchioles causing expulsion of material. Relaxing expectorants soothe bronchial spasm and loosen mucous secretions, helping in dry, irritating coughs.

Hepatics aid the liver. They tone, strengthen and in some cases increase the flow of bile. In a broad holistic approach to health they are of great importance because of the fundamental role of the liver in the working of the body.

Hypotensives are remedies that lower abnormally elevated blood pressure.

Laxatives stimulate bowel movements. Stimulating laxatives should not be used longterm. If this appears to be necessary then diet, general health and stress should all be closely considered.

Nervines help relieve the nervous system and can be meaningfully subdivided into three groups: Nervine tonics strengthen and restore the nervous system. Nervine relaxants ease anxiety and tension by soothing both body and mind. Nervine stimulants directly stimulate nerve activity.

Rubefacients generate a localized increase in blood flow when applied to the skin, helping healing, cleansing and nourishment. They are often used to ease the pain and swelling of arthritic joints.

Tonics nurture and enliven. Truly gifts of nature to a suffering humanity, tonics are whole plants that enliven whole human bodies, gifts of the Mother Earth to her children. To ask how they work is to ask how life works!

Vulneraries are remedies that promote wound healing. Used mainly to describe herbs for skin lesions, the action is just as relevant for inner wounds such as stomach ulcers.

For Further Reading

Books about Stress

Thomas L. Leaman, *Healing the Anxiety Diseases*. New York: Plenum Press, 1992.

Bob Whitmore, *Living with Stress and Anxiety: A Self-Help Guide*. Manchester University Press, 1987.

Benjamin Wolman and George Striker, eds., *Anxiety and Related Disorders: a Handbook*. Wiley, 1994.

John Mason, *Guide to Stress Reduction*. Celestial Arts, Berkeley, 1985.

Edmund Jacobson, *Progressive Relaxation*. Midway Reprint. University of Chicago Press, 1974.

Martha Davis, Elizabeth Robbins Eshelman and Matthew McKay, *The Relaxation and Stress Reduction Workbook*. New Harbinger Publications, Oakland, 1988.

Edmund J. Bourne, *The Anxiety and Phobia Workbook*. New Harbinger Publications, Oakland 1990.

Books about Herbal Medicine

Norman G. Bisset, (ed.) *Herbal Drugs & Phytopharmaceuticals*. CRC Press, Boca Raton, 1994.

Maude Grieve, *A Modern Herbal.* Volumes I and II, Dover Publications, New York, 1971.

David Hoffmann, *An Elder's Herbal.* Inner Traditions, Rochester, 1992.

David Hoffmann, *The Herbal Handbook.* Inner Traditions, Rochester, 1988.

David Hoffmann, *The Complete Illustrated Holistic Herbal.* Element Books, Shaftesbury, 1996.

Kathi Keville and Mindy Green, *Aromatherapy: A Complete Guide to the Healing Art.* Crossing Press, 1995.

Simon Mills, *Dictionary of Modern Herbalism.* Inner Traditions, Rochester, 1985.

Michael Murray and Joseph Pizzorno, *Encyclopedia of Natural Medicine.* Prime Publishing, Rocklin, 1990.

Michael Murray, *Stress, Anxiety and Insomnia.* Prime Publishing, Rocklin, 1995.

Rudolf Weiss, *Herbal Medicine.* Medicina Biologica, Portland, 1988.

Herbal Suppliers

Seeds

Abundant Life Seed Association, P.O. Box 772, 1029 Lawrence St., Port Townsend, WA 98368

Seeds of Change, PO Box 15700, Santa Fe, NM 87506-5700

Herbal Products

Eclectic Institute, 11231 SE Market St., Portland, OR 97216

Gaia Herbs, 62 Old Littleton Road, Harvard, MA 01451

HerbPharm, 347 East Fork Road, Williams, OR 97544

Herbalist & Alchemist Inc., P.O. Box 553, Broadway, NJ 08808, (908) 689-9020

Herbs Etc., 1340 Rubina Circle, Santa Fe, MN 87501

Nature's Way Products, 10 Mountain Springs Parkway, P.O. Box 2233, Springville, UT, 84663

Rainbow Light Nutritional Systems, 207 McPherson St., Santa Cruz, CA 95060

Simpler's Botanical, P.O. Box 39, Forestville, CA 95436

Traditional Medicinal Herb Tea Company, Sebastopol, CA 95472

Wind River, P.O. Box 3876, Jackson, WY 83001

Bulk Herbs

Blessed Herbs, 109 Barre Plains Road, Oakham, MA 01068

Frontier Cooperative Herbs, Box 299, Norway, IA 52318

Mountain Rose, P.O. Box 2000, Redway, CA 95560

Trinity Herbs, P.O. Box 199, Bodega, CA 94992

Pacific Botanicals, 4350 Fish Hatchery Rd., Grants Pass, OR 97527

Bibliography

Barenboim, G. M. and Kozlova, N.B. Use of Eleutherococcus extract for increasing the biological resistance of man exposed to different unfavourable environmental factors (A Review).

Brekhman, II, Kirillov, O. Effect of eleutherococcus on alarm-phase of stress. Life Sci 1969, Feb 1;8(3):113-21.

Ulrich, R. S. and R. F. Simons. Recovery from stress during exposure to everyday outdoor environments. In: J. Wineman, R. Barnes, and C. Zimring (eds.). The Costs of Not Knowing: Proceedings of the Seventeenth Annual Conference of the Environmental Design Research Association. Environmental Design Research Association, Washington, D.C. 1986.

Ulrich, R. S. View through a window may influence recovery from surgery. Science, 1984. 224:420-421.

"Treatment of mild/moderate depressions with hypericum," Harrer, G; Sommer, H. Phytomedicine. 1994 (1):3-8.

Natural Child Care Riggs, Maribeth. Harmony Books, New York, 1989.

Medicinal Valerian. Molodozhnikova, LM. Feldsher Akush 1988, Jan; 53(1):44-6 (Published in Russian).

INDEX